Medical Ethics and the Elderly
FOURTH EDITION

Edited by

GURCHARAN S RAI

Consultant Physician
Whittington Hospital, London

Foreword by
STEVE ILIFFE
Professor of Primary Care for Older People
University College London

Law sections edited by
GURDEEP S RAI

Illustrations by
IVA BLACKMAN

Radcliffe Publishing
London • New York

Radcliffe Publishing Ltd
St Mark's House
Shepherdess Walk
London N1 7BQ
United Kingdom

www.radcliffehealth.com

The paper used for the text pages of this book
is FSC® certified. FSC (The Forest Stewardship
Council®) is an international network to promote
responsible management of the world's forests.

Typeset by Darkriver Design, Auckland, New Zealand
Manufacturing managed by 21six

Contents

Foreword to the fourth edition

Modern medicine is uncomfortable because it is conflictual. Doctors struggle to contain the tensions arising from an ageing society, increasingly powerful therapies, cost-containment within services, medical consumerism, and legal and moral discourse about responsibility and blame.

The demographic transition means that demand for the care of disabled people – particularly the oldest old – outruns the supply of services designed for a different population, revealing the obsolescence of the UK health service. The complexity of older people with multiple disorders and deficits exceeds the capabilities of staff, who complain that they are the wrong sort of patient who should be elsewhere. And hospital wards filled with old, frail patients are daily reminders of depersonalisation, disability and death – the opposites of the curative model most doctors adhere to. The pastoral role that may be needed sits uncomfortably with the practitioners' repertoire of technical skills.

Ironically, the triumphs of modern medicine accentuate this problem of complexity, by treating heart disease effectively, improving survival after stroke, achieving cure in some cancers and refining surgical methods. We live longer, and accumulate our disabilities.

Health services funded from pooled budgets are necessarily utilitarian, seeking the greatest good for the greatest number, whilst practitioners are deontologists, focusing on the needs of the patient in front of them. Health services are increasingly industrialised, in an assembly line form that Henry Ford would recognise. Increasingly, decision-making is devolved whilst standard-setting is centralised. And everywhere there is cost-containment and pressure to innovate – that is, to redesign practice to make it more efficient and productive.

Patients exert pressure through medical consumerism, not simply by shopping around but through citizens' challenges to physician authority, expressed as demands, complaints and litigation. The transnational patient acquires medical opinions, investigations and treatments from their place of current residence, their cultural home and their community's diaspora. In super-diverse societies like those of Western Europe and North America, the basic assumptions individuals and families have about matters of life and death are varied but also changeable, as host and migrant cultures meet and modify each other.

Finally, the discourse of the law frames medical practice in new ways, defining rights and responsibilities through the Human Rights Act and protecting the interests of older people, in particular through the Mental Capacity Act (2005) and the Equality Act (2010). Moral discourse about compassion, dignity and blame saturates the NHS and is promoted by politicians, professional bodies and campaigning tabloid papers.

These pressures, combined in different ways, are felt in wards, outpatient clinics and GP surgeries every day. Practitioners learn how to manage them on the job, case by case, because learning ethics by numbers makes no sense. Hence this book, which combines a primer for the novice with advanced reasoning for the expert, both readerships being led through a range of very authentic case studies. The novice can look up the basic elements of current law, or acquire some rules of thumb about assessment of capacity or quality of life. The expert can think about clinical scenarios where there are no right answers, and all is contingent, or work out how the loss of the privilege of driving might be reframed to maximise mobility. Every practitioner should have this book, and it should be well-thumbed.

Professor Steve Iliffe
Professor of Primary Care for Older People
University College London
May 2014

Forewords to the third edition

Ten years in print and a new third edition of *Medical Ethics and the Elderly* is a cause for celebration. The book takes its place in the canon of Geriatric Medicine, earned because of its relevance and clear presentation of the complex moral issues. The third edition is reinvigorated by the addition of new younger authors who have upheld the tradition of concise incisive contributions informed by active engagement with clinical problems. The book retains its shape, style and length, resisting the temptation to expand the content beyond recognition. There is only one additional chapter 'Communication, barriers to it and information sharing' which is well written and thought provoking. Dr Gurcharan Rai has shown great skill in editing, incorporating the many changes in legislation that have occurred since the second edition while retaining the practicality and instructiveness of the text.

Medical ethics continues to grow in importance as a core subject in medical education. Those of us dealing with the old and vulnerable need to have skills in ethical reasoning and an up-to-date knowledge of the relevant legislation. This book more than achieves its aims of providing not only a practical guide but also a readable account of the principles and practice of ethics as they apply to the specialty of medicine for the elderly. It can be used both for reference and as a textbook from which the basic skills of ethical reasoning can be acquired. A must read book for anyone training in the specialty and an essential core text for every geriatrician's office.

The ethical challenges the medical profession face are becoming more demanding. The developments of high-tech interventions pose both benefits and risks to patients. The public are thankfully better informed and able to exert more influence on issues which were previously reserved to professionals. For example, there is a growing clamour for physician-assisted suicide in terminally ill patients which divides professional opinion. Doctors need to be able to react to the challenges in an informed professional manner that can only be achieved by them having the ethical literacy which is exemplified by the contents of this excellent book.

Doctors like certainty and medicine is easy when one can make decisions by simply following guidelines or protocols. Geriatrics is however probably the most complex branch of medicine. Most of our decisions fall in the grey area between black and white. In trying to make the best choices for patients, ethical considerations always play a part. Dr Gurchuran Rai exemplifies a careful and thoughtful approach to medicine and his achievement in editing three editions of this influential book, including his own original contributions, is to be greatly admired.

I unreservedly recommend this book. The new edition meets the requirements of today's practice and this and future editions will provide a core text for doctors and students for many years to come.

Jeremy Playfer MD FRCP
Emeritus Consultant, Royal Liverpool
and Broadgreen University Hospital
Honorary Clinical Lecturer, University of Liverpool
and Past President, British Geriatrics Society
May 2009

Since publication of the second edition of this book in 2004, the international phenomenon of rapid population aging has continued unabated. Similarly, the medical, ethical, legal, social and economic challenges accompanying this demographic development have grown, and continue to grow, increasingly numerous and complex. For example, in the United Kingdom over the past half decade, a panoply of legislative developments (including receipt of Royal Assent to The Mental Capacity Act in 2005) and organisational guidelines and codes pertaining to the ethical delivery of medical care to older individuals have emerged and are reflected in many parts of this new third edition.

Similarly, there has been a great amount of relevant legal and economic activity in recent years in the United States in response to the graying of its citizenry. Of course, important differences persist between the UK and the United States in terms of legal, social and economic climate, and those differences certainly may affect the ethics of providing – and paying for – healthcare for older persons in each country.

Nonetheless, there remain important commonalities in the basic values and tensions confronting medical caregivers for the aged in both nations. Generic ethical concerns that UK and American healthcare providers regularly confront (such as the need to delicately balance moral reverence for individual self-determination, on one hand, and society's simultaneous responsibility to maximise the older person's good and minimise harm, on the other) may be characterised by unique nuances in the geriatric arena. The special challenges involved in caring for the aged may result from particular factors inherent in this patient population (for example, a higher incidence and prevalence of cognitive and emotional impairment), the types of institutional and community settings within which geriatric services are provided, and the focus of geriatric care on the objectives of maximising the patient's ability to function well in daily life and achieve an optimal quality of life, rather than on simply extending the length of life.

In both the UK and the US, ethical decisions must be made and actions taken (or purposefully not taken) within distinct legal boundaries. Despite the legal superstructure in each jurisdiction, however, the ethical aspects of medical care remain for the most part self-enforcing. Thus, the various chapters in this book acknowledge that geriatric practice 'on the ground' (that is, in real life situations) is determined by healthcare provider virtues and patient wishes as much, if not more, than by academic ethics or legal edicts emanating from the legislature, government agency, or the judiciary.

This comprehensive and timely third edition should assist geriatric professionals to manage, in an ethically tolerable and perhaps even laudatory manner, circumstances entailing inconsistent and sometimes seemingly incompatible individual and institutional values. The chapter contributors do not pretend that there are objectively 'correct' answers to the dilemmas posed by an aging patient population, but they do make available to the reader – through the skillful employment of numerous hypothetical problems, among other effective methods of presentation – a very useful grounding upon which to build more-than-adequate applied ethical analyses of key concerns.

Differences in legal, social and economic climates notwithstanding, there is much that the UK and US aging services communities can teach to, and learn from, each other. Even more than its previous version, this thoroughly updated edition of *Medical Ethics and the Elderly* will not only assist physicians, medical students, and other healthcare providers in the UK regarding the ethical questions with which they regularly must deal, but will also facilitate cross-national pollination of ethical ideas and skills among healthcare practitioners on both sides of the Atlantic.

Marshall B Kapp JD, MPH, FCLM
Garwin Distinguished Professor of Law and Medicine
Southern Illinois University School of Law, USA
May 2009

Preface to the fourth edition

While the basic principles of medical ethics remain the same, since the publication of the third edition of this book in 2009 there have been changes made to the law and updates made to clinical guidance that have an impact on the clinical management of patients. These include:

➤ the Equality Act 2010, which maintains the right of older people to treatment without discrimination
➤ case law on withdrawing nutrition and hydration
➤ updated guidance on resuscitation from the Resuscitation Council (UK), the British Medical Association and the Royal College of Nursing
➤ redefining of good medical practice by the General Medical Council
➤ abolition of the Liverpool Care Pathway, with updated guidance on end-of-life care and advance care planning.

In addition to updating the chapters from the previous edition, this edition has two new chapters: Chapter 8, 'Testamentary capacity and the role of the physician', and Chapter 13, 'Religious beliefs of patients and end-of-life decisions'.

Despite these changes, however, the main aim of this book remains the same – it is intended to be a practical guide for medical staff, particularly trainees, and other professionals who are involved in making difficult clinical decisions during their day-to-day care of older persons and medical students.

Gurcharan S Rai
May 2014

Preface to the third edition

Since the publication of the second edition, the Mental Capacity Act 2005 received Royal Assent in 2005 and was implemented in two stages in 2007. This Act provides a comprehensive framework for decision making on behalf of adults who lack capacity to make decisions on their own behalf. In addition, there have been several other significant publications including:

➤ an update on consent from the General Medical Council in 2008
➤ a guide from the National Council for Palliative Care on advance decisions to refuse treatment
➤ a British Medical Association publication on end-of-life decisions in 2007
➤ guidance from the National Institute for Health and Clinical Excellence and the Social Care Institute for Excellence on supporting people with dementia and their carers in health and social care in 2006
➤ an update on decisions relating to cardiopulmonary resuscitation from the British Medical Association in 2007
➤ new guidance on confidentiality from the General Medical Council in 2004
➤ National Health Service Code of Practice on Confidentiality in 2005.

The updated chapters have included the provisions of the Mental Capacity Act and the above publications. In addition, we have included a new chapter on communication with older people. However, the main aim of the book remains the same – it is intended to be a practical guide for junior medical staff, including specialist registrars. Other professionals who are involved with doctors in making difficult decisions will also find this text useful, as will medical students who now have to learn about medical ethics and their application in day-to-day management of patients, as part of the undergraduate curriculum.

Gurcharan S Rai
May 2009

Preface to the second edition

Since the publication of the first edition of this book in 1999 we have seen the introduction of the Human Rights Act 1998, which incorporates the European Convention of Human Rights into UK law, the production of new guidelines on cardiopulmonary resuscitation by the British Medical Association in 2002, the new draft bill on mental incapacity, the new guidelines on consent for treatment and the publication of the National Service Framework for Older People, with a commitment to abolish ageism in clinical practice. The updated chapters have included these changes in law, the new guidelines and the new standards set out in the National Service Framework for Older People. In addition, two important new chapters on confidentiality and on ethical issues and driving have been added.

However, the main aim of the book remains the same – it is intended to be a practical guide for junior medical staff, including specialist registrars. Other professionals who are involved with doctors in making difficult decisions will also find this text useful, as will medical students who now have to learn about medical ethics and their application in day-to-day management of patients, as part of the undergraduate curriculum.

Gurcharan S Rai
March 2004

About the editor

Gurcharan S Rai is a consultant physician at the Whittington Hospital, London, and a member of the British Geriatrics Society and the Special Group on Medical Ethics. He is a Training Programme Director and Regional Advisor for Geriatric Medicine for the North East and Central regions of London.

List of contributors

Aza Abdulla
Geriatrician and Consultant Physician
Department of Elderly Care
Princess Royal University Hospital,
London

Jonathan Birns
Consultant in Stroke Medicine, Geriatrics
and General Medicine
Guy's and St Thomas' NHS Foundation
Trust, London

Iva Blackman
Consultant Physician and Geriatrician
USA

Ann Bowling
Professor of Health Sciences
Faculty of Health Sciences
University of Southampton
Southampton

Jim Eccles
Retired Consultant Physician in Geriatric
Medicine
St James's University Hospital, Leeds

Premila Fade
Consultant Geriatrician
Poole Hospital NHS Foundation Trust,
Dorset

Philippa Gee
Speech and Language Therapist
The Hampshire Hospitals Foundation
Trust
Basingstoke and North Hampshire
Hospital, Hampshire

Catherine Harvey
Consultant in Care of Elderly and Acute
Medicine
University College London Hospital NHS
Trust

Steven Luttrell
Consultant Physician in Older People's
Services
St Pancras Hospital, London
Medical Director
BUPA, London

David Oliver
Professor of Medicine for Older People
City University London, London

Desmond O'Neill
Professor of Medical Gerontology
Consultant Physician in Geriatric and
Stroke Medicine
Department of Medical Gerontology,
Trinity Centre for Health Sciences,
Adelaide and Meath Hospital, Dublin

Kamilla K Porter
General Practitioner
Rochford, Essex
Clinical Advisor and Sessional GP Lead
EQUIP (Education and Quality in
Primary Care), Essex

Gurdeep S Rai
Solicitor
London

David Robinson
Consultant Physician in Geriatric
Medicine
St James's Hospital, Dublin

Gwen M Sayers
Consultant Physician
London

Martin J Vernon
Consultant Physician in Elderly Medicine
Wythenshawe Hospital, Manchester

CHAPTER 1

Principles of medical ethics

Kamilla K Porter and Gurcharan S Rai

Medical knowledge and technology have advanced at a spectacular rate. This voyage of discovery has led to a wealth of ethical issues unimaginable to the original followers of the Hippocratic oath. Steeped in the history of philosophy and religion, the development of medical ethics has been an attempt to unravel and resolve the moral complexities and dilemmas that have faced doctors through the ages. Several tenets of medical ethics have survived to the modern day – for example, *primum non nocere* (first do no harm). Other concepts, such as the notion of communal responsibility and justice, have arisen in the complex modern medical era. When faced with an ethical dilemma, a useful starting point for critical reflection and decision-making is the 'four principles' model pioneered by the ethicists Beauchamp and Childress.[1] In their classic text *Principles of Biomedical Ethics*[1] they propose that at the heart of moral reasoning in healthcare lie the principles of *autonomy*, *justice*, *beneficence* and *non-maleficence*. This approach has met with some criticism as being too simplistic, but of great appeal is that these prima facie principles offer flexibility, represent a neutral frame of reference applicable to patients from different cultures and religions and are independent of political doctrines.[2]

There has been a proliferation of ethical guidelines from different medical professional bodies such as the General Medical Council, the Royal College of Nursing and medical defence organisations with regard to clinical practice, as well as local and national ethical codes with regard to research. It has been argued that merely a theoretical model of moral principles can no longer be used to resolve common ethical predicaments in modern healthcare, as in many cases the law stipulates what action is required. Consider the impact of the Human Rights Act 1998 on ethical decisions in healthcare – for example, article 2 (the right to life), article 3 (the right to freedom from inhuman and degrading treatment) and article 14 (the right to be free from discriminatory practices such as ageism), which affect policies relating to resuscitation orders, aspects of palliative care practice and the level of care in nursing homes.[3] In the UK, where healthcare is mainly provided by the National Health Service, the advent of the Care Quality Commission, the raft of recommendations in Don Berwick's report into patient safety,[4] and Robert Francis QC's report following the Mid Staffordshire tragedy,[5] which highlighted gross lapses of moral judgement, will also influence ethical decision-making.

As the media, including the Internet and expanding social media networks, have provided the public with greater access to information on medicine and health, the profile of patient autonomy has been raised further. The 'four principles' approach discussed in this introductory chapter does not serve as a manual with precise instructions, but rather it provides a framework with which to analyse ethical problems and guidelines. A useful way of thinking about the 'four principles' model is to consider each principle as one of the four nucleotides that constitute 'moral DNA', capable in combination or on their own of clarifying and justifying the general norms that underlie health-care ethics.[6]

AUTONOMY

Autonomy is about respecting patients' wishes and facilitating and encouraging their input into the medical decision-making process. The issue of informed consent and refusal lies at the heart of this principle. To respect a patient's autonomy is to give that individual a greater balance of power in the doctor–patient relationship. It entails explaining not only what is wrong with that person, but also the options and implications of any proposed investigation and treatment and the associated risks and benefits. The practitioner needs to provide the patient with as much information as he or she both wishes for and requires in order to make a decision.

Such information needs to be delivered in a clear and concise manner. A balance must be struck between confusing the individual with medical jargon and adopting an overly simplified approach that fails to include important details. The art of pitching the consultation at the right level is by no means straightforward, but where possible by ensuring that the patient understands his or her particular medical problem and management options the doctor should avoid the pitfall of using his or her own personal value system to judge what is best for the patient.

The issue of autonomy is all the more poignant among the elderly population in a society where older people can lose respect and personal choice. With its emphasis on patient-centred care and rooting out age discrimination, the National Service Framework for Older People[7] launched in 2001 promoted greater autonomy among the elderly, highlighting 'the need to view service users as active participants in, rather than subjects of, the care-providing process'.[7] Although designed as a 10-year programme, the original National Service Framework standards remain relevant and clinically valid and have been further developed – for example, the National Dementia Strategy.

The application of the principle of autonomy can be seen in the following case of an 80-year-old diabetic woman who was admitted to hospital with cardiac failure following a myocardial infarction. Her mental faculties were fully intact and she was making a steady recovery when her foot became ischaemic. Conservative management was instigated, but the foot could not be salvaged. The vascular surgeons explained on several occasions that in order to curtail the ascending ischaemia and to prevent potentially life-threatening infection, she needed a below-knee amputation. She was informed of her considerable anaesthetic risk, as well as the likelihood of remaining in hospital for several weeks after surgery and then needing a substantial care package. The patient requested time to talk to her family, and after further discussion with both the physicians and the surgeons she declined surgery. Over the ensuing days her leg became gangrenous and she died from overwhelming sepsis. The case sparked differing viewpoints among the medical staff, some of who felt that with the option of local anaesthetic block instead of a general anaesthetic, it was worth risking surgery to prevent this hitherto active and independent individual dying from sepsis. Others felt that with dedicated nursing care and good pain control, the patient's refusal to go ahead with surgery was preferable to a long and complicated recovery period and loss of her independent lifestyle.

This case scenario illustrates how, when management options are no longer clear-cut, the patient can play a pivotal role in guiding the doctor through an ethical maze. The principle of autonomy, although a noble ideal, is not without its limitations. Patients may be unable to contribute fully to discussions about their care for a variety of reasons – for example, in an emergency situation when swift intervention is needed, or when there are communication difficulties that could be due to cultural and language barriers or practical problems such as impairment after a stroke. Furthermore, some patients may reject opportunities to exercise their autonomy and request that the doctor acts on their behalf, as is evident in the statement 'whatever you think best, doctor'. Under such circumstances the doctor may have to decide on the most appropriate course of action, but only after he or she has given that patient the option of sharing in the decision-making process.

Doctors themselves may feel threatened and challenged by involving patients in making decisions about treatment – for example, because of time constraints in a busy clinic or surgery and a lack of appropriate information to support patients' decisions. Some doctors may feel uncomfortable and lack the skills to negotiate a decision with the patient.[8] This is an area of ongoing research and one that has implications for medical training. It has been argued that failing to accommodate patients' needs and preferences will ultimately diminish doctors' standing.[9]

Respecting autonomy becomes more complicated in cases of mental incompetence. Deciding how to treat the elderly woman with the ischaemic foot would have been more difficult if she had also been suffering from dementia. In such situations the doctor is obliged to look beyond the individual in the sickbed and to consider the patient in the context of her home and family – in other words, taking into account quality-of-life issues. Other health professionals, family members and carers can provide invaluable information. The patient may have made her wishes clear to relatives before her mental deterioration, or appointed an attorney under the lasting power of attorney or in the form of an advance decision/advance decision to refuse treatment. The ethical reverberations of mental incompetence and the issues of advance decision/advance decision to refuse treatment and quality-of-life measurements are examined in detail in later chapters.

JUSTICE

In the context of healthcare, justice implies an impartial and fair approach to treatment and the distribution of resources. Doctors discriminate unfairly if they allow their prejudices to directly influence their professional work. Established ethical and human rights codes condemn any form of discrimination on the grounds of age, race, sex, religion or sexual orientation. The General Medical Council's *Good Medical Practice*[10] stresses that doctors must not allow any personal views about patients to prejudice their assessment of the patient's clinical needs or delay or restrict the patient's access to care. Furthermore, as a result of the Equality Act 2010, it is now unlawful for National Health Service and social care service providers and professionals to discriminate, victimise or harass a person because of his or her age.[11]

A much-debated topic is whether to continue to provide unrestricted healthcare to individuals whose lifestyle choices and behaviour have contributed to their ill health – for example, smoking, intravenous drug use and obesity. If despite appropriate advice and information about the dangers of high-risk activities such as smoking a patient continues to take that risk, accepting his or her decision is effectively taking into account that patient's autonomy. At the same time, encouraging the patient to take responsibility for his or her medical problems is also to respect that patient's autonomy.

However, as the cost of healthcare continues to spiral, the issue of social justice and the needs of other health service users cannot be overlooked. Would it be fair to withhold treatment for those who engage in voluntary risk-taking at the expense of their health? There are no easy answers to this question, and it is difficult to attribute an individual's ill health solely to his or her personal actions, as genetic, environmental and social factors can also play a role. Furthermore, some risk-taking can result in fewer rather than more healthcare costs, as such individuals may die earlier and more quickly than those who engage in a less risky lifestyle.

A caring society demands that limited resources are allocated in a just manner. The *Oxford Dictionary of Philosophy* defines distributive justice as 'the link between a distributive system and the maximisation of well-being'. Difficulties arise because of the inevitable scarcity of resources and subsequent conflicts between competing specialty groups. Increasingly, health professionals and governments are confronted with legitimate competing concerns and have to acknowledge the prioritisation of patient needs. When a potential treatment is wanted for a patient, the final decision may be that because of the overwhelming need of others, the purchasing of this expensive treatment cannot be justified. In recent years numerous national and local clinical guidelines have emerged that outline the rationale for denying certain treatments, and a difficult balance has to be struck between personal autonomy and the benefit to society at large. This is an area that regularly engenders differences of opinion among patients and their advocates, clinicians, healthcare managers and politicians.

In an era of increasing healthcare costs, an ageing population and development of more sophisticated treatments and procedures, the issue of healthcare rationing cannot be avoided. Central to this issue are questions of what we mean by human dignity and what level of basic care can still be deemed humane. Setting and defining the limits of an acceptable level of minimum medical care is a dynamic process that requires input from medical professionals, politicians, health managers and the general public. It has been argued that at the very least the aim of basic healthcare is to prevent premature death, to enable an individual to function as a productive member of society and, when that is no longer possible, to alleviate distressing symptoms for the remaining duration of that individual's life and as he or she approaches death.[12]

BENEFICENCE AND NON-MALEFICENCE

The doctor should act to promote the welfare of his or her patient and to do good (beneficence). An action that is taken to benefit the patient may entail risks, so at the same time we have to consider the principle of non-maleficence (avoiding doing harm). In essence we are looking at a cost–benefit ratio, and it is of critical importance that it is patient centred. Acting in the best interests of the patient is a stance that also incorporates respecting autonomy, and conflicts can arise between these principles. Consider the patient who requests an investigation or treatment that the doctor finds to be unwarranted clinically – for example, a lumbar spine X-ray for an episode of mild lower back pain. The doctor's refusal could be seen as paternalistic, and the patient may feel aggrieved, but the doctor has to weigh up the risks and merits of the intervention requested against the patient's wishes and the preservation of a good doctor–patient relationship.

Sometimes the risk of harm to others in the population needs to be taken into account, and the principle of non-maleficence may outweigh the patient's autonomy. An example would be the detention in hospital of a patient who has pulmonary tuberculosis and has repeatedly failed to take his or her medication regularly in the community. Such drastic action has been deemed ethical on the grounds of the infective risk that the patient poses to the public, and the possibility that the patient could develop multi-drug resistance and become more unwell through his or her haphazard use of medication.

Deciding what is beneficial overall to the patient and what constitutes harm can be fraught with difficulty, particularly with regard to end-of-life decisions such as withholding or withdrawing treatment and the much-debated issue of euthanasia and physician-assisted suicide. The notion of saving life underpins medical training. However, nowadays there is also a greater emphasis on examining the quality of life and the concept of dignified death. In the UK, where euthanasia is illegal, doctors follow the doctrine of double effect, under which it is permissible to administer medication to alleviate distressing symptoms of terminal illness even though the patient may die sooner as a result, but the doctor has to prove that the objective is to relieve suffering, not to shorten life. The fear is that if doctors actively assisted patients in ending their lives, the door would be opened to a slippery slope towards involuntary euthanasia, where the old or frail might be put under pressure by relatives or be made to feel like an unwanted burden to their families and society. Some argue that there is a very thin line between respecting a terminally ill patient's refusal of life-sustaining treatment and yet turning down their request for assistance in directly ending their life in order to avoid more suffering.[13] These topics will be explored further in later chapters.

CONCLUSION

Healthcare professionals require an ethical basis for their day-to-day work. The 'four principles' model outlined in this chapter has its limitations and may not necessarily provide obvious answers, but it is a useful tool to identify and help in the analysis of ethical dilemmas.

From doing something seemingly straightforward such as performing a blood test to completing 'do not attempt resuscitation' orders, doctors make ethical decisions – taking into account the patient's wishes (respecting his or her autonomy), weighing up the benefits against the possible harm of any medical action (beneficence and non-maleficence) and taking into consideration whether that action and its cost are fair overall (exercising justice).

The onus of such decision-making no longer rests with the doctor alone. Increasingly, it is a multidisciplinary team that delivers healthcare, with the views of all those on the team being instrumental in influencing the outcome for a patient. Furthermore, social media, websites, television, newspapers and patient groups now provide the public with information about medicine and health on an unprecedented scale. This trend, together with the passing of the Human Rights Act 1998, has brought the issue of patient autonomy to even greater prominence. In addition, the rapid changes in modern medicine, ongoing research and increasing specialisation mean that ethical decision-making requires the engagement not only of the patient and healthcare professionals but also of society at large.

REFERENCES

1. Beauchamp TL, Childress JF. *Principles of Biomedical Ethics.* 7th ed. New York, NY: Oxford University Press; 2013.
2. Gillon R. Medical ethics: four principles plus attention to scope. *BMJ.* 1994; **309**(6948): 184–8.
3. Hewson B. Why the Human Rights Act matters to doctors. *BMJ.* 2000; **321**(7264): 780–1.
4. National Advisory Group on the Safety of Patients in England. A promise to learn – a commitment to act: Improving the safety of patients in England. *Berwick Review into Patient Safety.* London: Department of Health; 2013. Available at: www.gov.uk/government/uploads/system/uploads/attachment_data/file/226703/Berwick_Report.pdf (accessed 2 April 2014).
5. Francis, R. *The Mid Staffordshire NHS Foundation Trust Public Inquiry.* London: The Mid Staffordshire NHS Foundation Trust Public Inquiry; 2010. Available at: www.midstaffspublicinquiry.com (accessed 24 March 2014).
6. Gillon R. Ethics needs principles—four can encompass the rest—and respect for autonomy should be "first among equals". *J Med Ethics.* 2003; **29**(5): 307–12.
7. *National Service Framework: older people.* London: Department of Health; 2001. Available at: www.gov.uk/government/publications/quality-standards-for-care-services-for-older-people (accessed 24 March 2014)
8. Say RE, Thomson R. The importance of patient preferences in treatment decisions: challenges for doctors. *BMJ.* 2003; **327**(7414): 542–5.
9. Coulter A. Patients' views of the good doctor. *BMJ.* 2002; **325**(7366): 668–9.
10. General Medical Council. *Good Medical Practice (2013).* Manchester: GMC; 2013. Available at: www.gmc-uk.org/guidance/good_medical_practice.asp
11. NHS Choices. *Equality and Diversity in the NHS.* London: NHS; 2012. Available at: www.nhs.uk/NHSEngland/thenhs/equality-and-diversity (accessed 24 March 2014).
12. Baillie HM, McGeehan JM, Garrett TM, *et al. Health Care Ethics.* 6th ed. Boston, MA: Pearson; 2012.
13. Doyal L, Doyal L. Why active euthanasia and physician assisted suicide should be legalised. *BMJ.* 2001; **323**(7321): 1079–80.

FURTHER READING AND USEFUL WEBSITES

- British Medical Association. *Ethics.* London: BMA; n.d. Available at: http://bma.org.uk/practical-support-at-work/ethics (accessed 24 March 2014).
- British Medical Association. *Medical Ethics Today: the BMA's handbook of ethics and law.* 3rd ed. Chichester: Wiley-Blackwell; 2012.
- General Medical Council: www.gmc-uk.org
- *Journal of Medical Ethics*: http://jme.bmj.com
- UK Clinical Ethics Network: www.ukcen.net

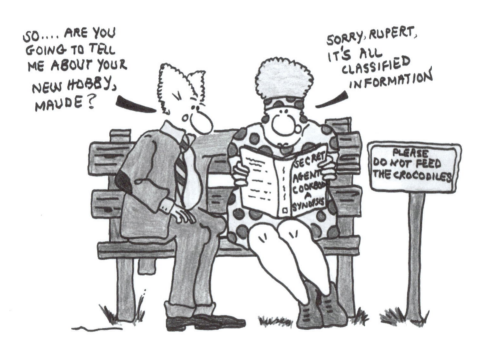

CHAPTER 2

Confidentiality

Catherine Harvey and Gurcharan S Rai

Confidentiality is one of the basic premises of medical practice and was enshrined in the Hippocratic oath:

> Whatever, in connection with my professional practice or not in connection with it, I see or hear, in the life of men, which ought not to be spoken of abroad, I will not divulge, as reckoning that all such should be kept secret.

Confidentiality is fundamental to the relationship between doctor and patient. Patients expect information they give to their doctors to be confidential, but they also expect good communication between health professionals. This chapter discusses the importance of confidentiality and sharing information with consent, and it outlines when information may be shared without consent and the consequences of doing this.

The protection of confidentiality has its basis in law, in professional codes of practice and in medical ethics.[1] In the UK, the General Medical Council's (GMC's) guidance on confidentiality states that doctors have a duty to respect the privacy of patients and to protect information given to them in confidence.[2] Any information obtained in a professional capacity is subject to this. Doctors must protect information and make sure that patients are aware of how it is used. Consent should always be obtained before sharing this information with others, unless there are exceptional circumstances. As well as a duty of care to an individual, doctors have a duty to the community at large. This, coupled with the nature of information shared between doctors and their patients, can lead to conflicts of interest. When these conflicts of interest occur and the question of disclosing information without consent arises, there must be clear ethical and legal justification for doing so. The GMC's guidance sets professional standards of practice, and although it is not legally binding, the courts take it seriously. Much of the legal requirement for confidentiality has developed from case law but it is also laid down in statute. The Data Protection Act 1998 provides a framework outlining how information should be processed, stored and shared and it gives an individual right of access to data held. The Human Rights Act 1998 protects the privacy of individuals by article 8 (the right to private and family life).

THE IMPORTANCE OF CONFIDENTIALITY

The need for confidentiality is based on two principles:
1. the patient's right to privacy and autonomy
2. the preservation of a doctor–patient relationship that is based on mutual trust.

We choose carefully the information that we share with others. This information helps us to shape our identity – how we view ourselves, how we want others to see us and, to an extent, how others perceive us. Patients share sensitive information with their doctors about their physical, emotional, social and sexual health that they may not share with anyone else. The assumption of confidentiality means that they can do this without fear of embarrassment or disapproval. Without an implicit understanding that information will be kept private, patients may feel unable to talk to their doctor openly and frankly. Any barrier to open communication could make the already challenging task of appropriate investigation and therapy even more difficult. The fears of HIV and AIDS patients in the 1980s and 1990s illustrated the potential wide-ranging consequences of compromising confidentiality. There are implications for an individual's personal relationships, work and finance, as well as the possibility of discrimination.

In reality, the public's perception of what confidentiality means and the practice of modern medicine may differ significantly. This is partly because of the increasing numbers of people involved in providing medical care. It is particularly true when caring for older patients. Those involved can range from nursing staff and physiotherapists to social workers, carers and day hospital receptionists. It is unlikely that patients are aware of the extent to which personal information is disseminated. There has also been an expansion in those who are not directly involved in patient care but who are involved in research and administration. IT systems such as electronic health records or national databases can also be seen to threaten our traditional idea of confidentiality. Organisations should make information readily available to patients explaining how information about them is shared and used.

Perhaps more pertinent for the majority of patients is how we deal with sensitive information in a busy general practice, emergency department or hospital ward. Patients may be asked to disclose what may be considered private information in a queue at reception at a general practice. On a hospital ward, patient care may be discussed within earshot of other patients or their relatives. Life-changing discussions, such as breaking bad news, are conducted with just a curtain separating the patient from the outside world. Indiscretion and carelessness are arguably the commonest forms of breaches of confidentiality. This may take the form of leaving notes open and unattended at a workstation, gossiping, or talking about patients in a hospital canteen. Lapses can also occur when we are caring for older people who are very frail or with whom we find it difficult to communicate – for example, because of deafness or dysarthria. We may find it simpler to talk to their next of kin. More detailed information is sometimes revealed to relatives and carers than to a patient, without having ensured the patient's consent.

In the UK the principle of confidentiality is not considered absolute. It is not always possible to obtain consent to share personal information. This can occur in an emergency situation where it is not practical to do so, or when patients decide to withhold consent or do not have the capacity to give it. The GMC guidance outlines when doctors are required to disclose information or when it can be justified.[2] These situations can be summarised as follows:
1. with the patient's consent
2. in the public interest
3. for the purposes of research and other secondary uses
4. when it is required by law.

Every attempt should be made to obtain consent. In the exceptional cases where this is not possible, the patient should be told of the decision, unless this will put individuals at risk or it undermines the purpose of disclosure.[2] Doctors should be prepared to justify any such decision. The circumstances and discussions should be carefully recorded. It is advisable to discuss the matter with a colleague or a professional body before arriving at such a decision.

SHARING INFORMATION WITH THE PATIENT'S CONSENT
Consent must be obtained before disclosing information to another party, unless there are exceptional circumstances. It is good practice to document this consent. Depending on the nature of the information being shared, this can be done formally with the patient's written consent or as a written record that verbal consent has been given. To give his or her consent, the patient should understand the nature and effects of the disclosure and have the capacity to make the decision.

It is essential that information is passed between health professionals to provide good healthcare. Clearly it is not always necessary to obtain explicit consent for this, provided that the patient has agreed to investigation or treatment. For instance, if a patient agrees to a specialist referral from his or her general practitioner (GP), then it is implied that the patient is happy for the GP to pass on details to the specialist. Patients expect health professionals to communicate effectively, and poor communication is a common source of frustration and complaints. However, difficulties can arise when patients and their doctors differ in their understanding of what information needs to be communicated and to whom. Only information that is relevant and required for optimum care should be disclosed, and it is the doctor's duty to ensure that the patient understands what information will be given. A doctor should also make sure that anyone receiving such information recognises that it is given in confidence.

If information is to be shared with others who are not involved in the healthcare of a patient, such as an employer, insurance company or benefits agency, then the patient's express consent must be obtained.[2] It is the doctor's responsibility to ensure that the patient understands what information is shared and any adverse effects that this may have. Consent should be in writing prior to sharing information and only factual, relevant information should be imparted. A copy of the report should be given to the patient before disclosing it to others, unless this would cause serious harm to an individual or breach another person's confidentiality. If a patient withholds consent then information can only be given if there is a legal requirement to do so or if it is in the public's interest,[2] as discussed later in this chapter.

Doctors have a duty to take part in clinical audit. All audit activities should conform to the requirements of the *NHS Confidentiality Code of Practice*,[3] which states that 'patients must be made aware that the information they give may be

---

CASE 2.1

Mrs J is an active 87-year-old. She is admitted as an emergency with abdominal pain. Investigation reveals a metastatic malignancy and treatment will be palliative. Mrs J insists that she does not want her family to be told. She says that she does not want her family worrying and feeling sorry for her and she wants to 'enjoy what is left' of her life. She has a caring family who have been fully informed of events until this point, and they now want to know what is wrong with Mrs J.

Comment

Mrs J's wishes must be respected. It may help to explore the reasons for her decision and the consequences for her, her family and the practicalities of her care. She may find it difficult to carry the burden of illness alone and to make plans without the assistance of her family. In the future a number of healthcare professionals such as district nurses or a palliative care team may be involved in her care. Information can only be passed on to others and referrals made with her consent. At some stage in her illness it is almost inevitable that she will need and want to inform her family, but she should decide when this will be. Her medical team should support her in this and she may value your support in talking to her family at a later time. Until then, you need to identify from Mrs J what information she would like her family to have and discussions with them will need to be handled delicately. It is important that all those involved in her care are aware of her views and that is clearly documented, to avoid any inadvertent breach of confidentiality, challenging as this may be.

recorded, may be shared in order to provide them with care, and may be used to support clinical audit.' The National Health Service Act 2006[4] makes provision for the collection of identifiable data for the purposes of clinical audit once patients have been informed. However, best practice is for the clinical audit data to be anonymous, unless there is a compelling reason for this to not be anonymous.

SHARING INFORMATION IN THE PUBLIC INTEREST

Information may be shared in the public interest. This can be to prevent the spread of infectious disease, to protect against serious harm or crime, or for medical research and other secondary uses.[2] Where possible, consent should be gained, but sometimes it is necessary to do this without consent. When making a decision to share information without consent, the potential benefits of making a disclosure need to be carefully weighed against the harm caused to the patient and the loss of faith in the medical profession for that patient and for others. We do not practise medicine in a vacuum and on occasion the public good will prevail. The definition of serious harm is a grey area, but the *NHS Confidentiality Code of Practice*[3] suggests it includes murder, manslaughter, rape or cases where individuals have suffered serious harm. Decisions where there is conflict between the rights of known individuals and of others are most challenging when the degree of harm and the probability of harm are hard to quantify. In these situations, attempts should be made to persuade the

---

CASE 2.2

Mr D has been diagnosed with early dementia. He looks after his wife, who is disabled following a stroke. Mr D tells his GP that he relies on his car to do the shopping and to take his wife out on trips that are important for their quality of life. You are concerned that Mr D may no longer be safe behind the wheel. You tell him he must contact the Driver and Vehicle Licensing Agency (DVLA) and tell them of his diagnosis. He insists that he will not do this because he must be allowed to continue driving. You judge that Mr D has capacity to make this decision.

Comment

The DVLA has clear requirements.[5] Dementia is one of the diagnoses they must be informed of. If Mr D is not deemed safe to drive, there is a risk to him and his wife and also to the public. He is legally obliged to tell the DVLA of his diagnosis. His doctor should tell him this and that the DVLA will not automatically revoke his licence on the basis of the diagnosis alone. If he still refuses to inform the DVLA, then it is the duty of his doctor to inform them. Mr D should be made aware of this.

patient to share information voluntarily or to give his or her consent, unless this would put people at risk. It might be helpful to ask the patient hypothetically what he or she would do if in the doctor's position. When information is shared without consent only relevant information should be divulged and the patient should be informed if it is practical and safe to do so. For patients who are unable to give consent because they lack capacity to do so, decisions must be made in accordance with the Mental Capacity Act 2005.

CASE 2.3

Mr W is a 75-year-old who has been admitted to hospital with a chest infection and falls. He is thin and unkempt and has a number of bruises on his arms and chest. He lives with his son and relies on him for help with getting washed and dressed, to prepare meals and do his cleaning and shopping. When the son has visited the ward, he has smelt of alcohol. Nurses raise the possibility of abuse and think that you should inform social services or the police. Mr W denies any problems at home and says that he wants to go home to his son.

Comment

Elder abuse can take the form of physical, emotional, sexual or financial abuse or neglect. There are no specific laws in the UK to protect the elderly from these forms of abuse; they are subject to the same laws as other, younger adults. Mr W is dependent on a close family member who may or may not be guilty of neglect or abuse. However, Mr W remains a competent adult capable of making his own decisions and he has the right to determine what information he shares with others. It would be wise to suggest supportive measures for Mr W and his son. The introduction of a care package may help to reduce stress on the family. It will provide a point of contact with external services, should Mr W need assistance. Any decision to breach confidentiality in such an instance needs to take into account the risk of serious harm to the individual or others, the vulnerability of the individual and the nature and impact of abuse. If Mr W lacked capacity to make these judgements, then further action would be needed to safeguard him. Institutions involved in the care of vulnerable adults should have a policy outlining the process that should be undertaken when abuse is suspected.

SHARING INFORMATION FOR RESEARCH AND OTHER NON-CLINICAL PURPOSES

Information obtained in clinical practice is used for other purposes, including medical research, education or training and public health or epidemiology.[2] These do not directly benefit an individual patient but are of use to society as a whole – for example, in improving patient safety or in health planning. While sharing much of this kind of information poses little threat to an individual, it has still been imparted in confidence, and the use and protection of such data has been controversial. Many patients will not be aware that information is used in this manner and consent should not be assumed. In broad terms, information should only be given to those who are bound by a duty of confidentiality, consent should be sought to share information and data should be anonymous. Research ethics committees ensure that research proposals are robust and take confidentiality into account. Each health organisation also has a Caldicott guardian. A Caldicott guardian's role is to protect the confidentiality of information and to ensure lawful and ethical information sharing. Identifiable information for secondary uses may be disclosed in limited circumstances without consent: if it is in the public interest, if it is required by law or if it is approved under section 251 of the National Health Service Act 2006.[2]

CASE 2.4

Mrs B's family comes to visit her in hospital. They hear a group of medical students on the ward discussing their mother's case with a junior doctor. Mrs B and her family are angry.

Comment

The value of confidentiality needs to be impressed upon medical students and other trainee health professionals from an early stage of their training. Most patients recognise the importance of medical education and are keen to assist in it. In any healthcare setting where medical students are learning, their presence and role should be made clear to patients. This includes GP consultations, clinics and ward rounds. If the students have already been involved in assessments of Mrs B, such as on a ward round, then she should already have been asked for permission for their involvement. Otherwise, the doctor and students should have gained consent to discuss the patient with medical students, as they would before taking a history or examining a patient. Subsequent teaching should have taken place in an area where Mrs B's confidentiality was protected and not where others could hear.

Increasing amounts of data are being stored on electronic systems such as national databases and electronic health records. Publicity surrounding the loss of information by other public bodies has led to concern about how information is stored and protected and how it can be accessed. The Data Protection Act 1998 safeguards information, whether it is held in paper form, electronically or in another medium such as pictures. On a day-to-day basis, it is important that users take the same care with computer records as they would with medical notes. This means not leaving screens unattended, remembering to log off and not sharing passwords. Particular care should be taken with portable storage devices and laptops.

SHARING INFORMATION WHEN REQUIRED TO BY LAW

In a court of law, a judge can order the disclosure of information. A doctor can object if he or she believes that the information is irrelevant but the decision falls to the judge. Information should not be given to either lawyers or police without express consent, unless justifiable as being in the public interest or required by law.[2] In these instances it may be prudent to consult with a medical defence organisation.

Information must also be disclosed if there is a statutory obligation to do so. This is the case in notifiable communicable diseases. Certain regulatory bodies – for example, those monitoring standards of care or fitness to practise – also have statutory rights to information. Again it is good practice to gain consent to share information if this is practicable.

SHARING INFORMATION IN PATIENTS WHO ARE UNABLE TO GIVE CONSENT

Doctors caring for older people will commonly look after those who lack capacity to consent to sharing information. This lack of capacity is most often due to dementia. When this occurs, health professionals must act in accordance with the Mental Capacity Act 2005 (England and Wales) or the Adults with Incapacity (Scotland) Act 2000, as discussed in Chapter 7, 'Mental capacity and best interests'. This means that those involved must act in the best interests of the patient, taking into account any known, previously expressed views or beliefs of the patient. Sharing clinical information can be especially important in this patient group. They may have complex medical problems and care needs. Important decisions regarding care, such as those surrounding artificial feeding or end-of-life care, may have been made and should be effectively communicated to provide a high standard of care.

Most often a patient's next of kin will act on his or her behalf and may be able to provide insight into a patient's values and beliefs to help in making decisions. A patient may have appointed a lasting power of attorney and so the attorney can do this. In the absence of a suitable family member or friend, an independent mental capacity advocate may be appointed (in England and Wales) by the local authority. This advocate should be provided with the necessary information to help patients and those caring for them to come to decisions. Patients should be supported to take part in the process as much as possible.

If an individual who lacks capacity does not want information to be shared but it is in his or her best interests to do so, then you may divulge that information, provided this is proportionate. Again it is important to document these discussions and to inform the patient. If capacity to make decisions is thought likely to fluctuate or if a patient may regain capacity then decisions should be postponed if possible.

CASE 2.5

The daughter of a patient with advanced dementia visits a hospital ward and asks for a medical update on her mother's condition and discharge plan. The doctor has known the patient for some time and is surprised not to have met this daughter before but answers her questions. The following day the patient's son expresses concern that information has been given to the patient's daughter. The relationship between mother and daughter had broken down many years ago and they had been estranged.

Comment

In this case the patient was unable to give consent. Sharing information is important but the rights to privacy and confidentiality of vulnerable individuals need to be upheld. However, it is reasonable to assume that patients would want information to be shared with those closest to them, unless they have stated otherwise.[2] Ideally, patients' views should be determined when they have capacity, but usually this does not occur. Complex family dynamics can cause dilemmas in patient care and it can be difficult to balance appropriate sharing of information with respect for privacy. In this case, provided the information from the son is correct, it is unlikely that the patient would have wanted information to be shared with her daughter.

SHARING INFORMATION FOLLOWING A DEATH

CASE 2.6

The nephew of an 89-year-old Greek patient who had attended the clinic for investigations in the past makes an appointment to see the doctor. The patient, his aunt, died 6 months ago and he is contesting her will, in which she left her estate to her brother. The nephew suspects that this will does not represent the wishes of his aunt, for it is written in English and her English was poor. He asks for copies of medical records showing that his aunt could not communicate well in English and that at each outpatient visit an interpreter was required.

Comment

Good communication with bereaved families is very important. However, even after a patient has died a doctor still has a duty of confidentiality. Doctors should not disclose any information if the patient has requested non-disclosure and this is documented in the medical records. While records for living patients are protected by the Data Protection Act 1998, the records of deceased patients are governed by the Access to Health Records Act 1990. The deceased's personal representative has the right to access the patient's medical records. This representative is the executor of the patient's will and is not necessarily the patient's next of kin. Others who have a claim arising out of a patient's death may also have access to records. In this instance, it is advisable to seek legal advice. There are circumstances where information must be shared after a patient's death. These include providing accurate information for death certificates or the coroner and when required by law, in the public interest or under section 251 of the National Health Service Act 2006.[2]

KEY POINTS

- Doctors have a duty to keep confidential any information that is learned in a professional capacity.
- There is a legal responsibility to protect confidentiality. This is based on case law and statute including the Data Protection Act 1998 and the Human Rights Act 1998. In the UK the General Medical Council lays down professional standards of practice for doctors.
- Consent must be obtained to share information. Patients should be aware of the extent of information shared and with whom it is shared. Information may also be shared if it is in the public interest, when required to by law or for the purpose of medical research or secondary uses.
- Breaches of confidentiality are most often unintentional or careless – for example, discussing a patient with a colleague in a lift, leaving notes or computer records unattended on a ward, talking to relatives without a patient's consent.
- Careful consideration must be given to sharing information in the absence of consent and it must be justifiable legally and ethically. Patients should be informed unless there is a good reason not to do so. Doctors must be prepared to justify these decisions. If in doubt, seek advice.
- In broad terms, for the purposes of medical research, education and public health, information should only be given to those who are bound by a duty of confidentiality, consent should be sought to share information and data should be anonymous.
- The duty of confidentiality persists after the death of a patient and medical records should only be shared with his or her personal representative.

REFERENCES

1. Mason JK, Laurie GT. Medical confidentiality. In: Mason JK, Laurie GT. *Mason and McCall Smith's Law and Medical Ethics.* 8th ed. Oxford: Oxford University Press; 2011. pp. 185–224.
2. General Medical Council. *Confidentiality.* Manchester: GMC; 2009. Available at: www.gmc-uk.org/static/documents/content/Confidentiality_0513_Revised.pdf (accessed 4 December 2013).
3. Department of Health. *NHS Confidentiality Code of Practice.* London: DH; 2003. Available at: www.gov.uk/government/uploads/system/uploads/attachment_data/file/200146/Confidentiality_-_NHS_Code_of_Practice.pdf (accessed 4 December 2013).
4. *National Health Service Act 2006 (c.41).* London: TSO; 2006. Available at: www.legislation.gov.uk/ukpga/2006/41/pdfs/ukpga_20060041_en.pdf (accessed 24 March 2014).
5. Drivers Medical Group, Driver and Vehicle Licensing Agency. *For Medical Practitioners: at a glance guide to the current medical standards of fitness to drive.* Swansea: DVLA; 2013. Available at: www.gov.uk/government/uploads/system/uploads/attachment_data/file/258991/aagv1.pdf (accessed 24 March 2014).

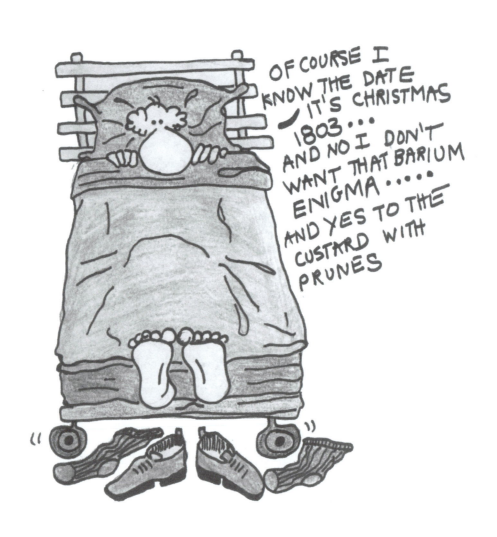

CHAPTER 3

Informed consent

Martin J Vernon

INTRODUCTION

Traditionally the process of making healthcare decisions has been articu-lated in terms of a contractual negotiation between health workers and their patients. Patients have a fundamental right to make choices about proposed healthcare interventions. This is based on the available information about anticipated benefits and harms of that intervention. It is also contingent upon their ability to make the decision at hand: broadly, their capacity to take in and weigh the information provided to them and to express their choices.

While this approach to consent is aligned to legal frameworks, which oper-ate in much of the developed world, its apparent simplicity, originating in the principle of respect for autonomy, poses a challenge to those involved in delivering care to vulnerable people in present-day society. Legal frameworks have at times struggled to keep pace with technological, economic and politi-cal developments in health and social care, sometimes leaving practitioners uncertain as to how to proceed. Now more than ever, the values and guiding principles that underpin good consent practice are of key importance to all involved in facilitating health and social care decisions for older people.

Patient choice is fundamental to the delivery of good healthcare practice.[1] Who would contemplate forcing treatment on an individual against his or her wishes or without seeking his or her views? This view of consent is accessible and based on the value of protecting individuals from unwanted interference. Arguably, however, it is also too narrow to accommodate the range of decision-making required in modern health and social care practice. It presupposes a range of choice with clearly defined outcomes in an environment of certainty. It appears to neglect the reality of modern health and social care where choices are restricted not just by clinicians but by economics or policy, and outcomes are at times diffuse, multiple and clouded by uncertainty.

In the last few decades much has been made of the rhetoric of 'person-centred' care.[2] Older people, particularly those with cognitive impairment, are sometimes by default excluded from making choices about their care in ways that may be considered mistreatment or abuse.[3] In recent times there has been positive and sustained policy shift towards placing people at the centre of their care decisions.[4] However, despite the rhetoric, recent times have also demonstrated that patient-centred choice is not universal. In England the Mid Staffordshire NHS Foundation Trust Public Inquiry cited many examples of poor care, which stemmed from neglect of the fundamental principle of choice.[5] In 2013 the UK government-commissioned review of the Liverpool Care Pathway for the Dying[6] also cited examples of patient (and family) exclusion from choices relating to fundamental aspects of patient care at the end of life, including resuscitation and other potentially life-sustaining or life-saving interventions. While the causative factors that underlie these examples are complex, at least two common themes have emerged: poor communication and uncertainty about outcome.

Increasingly, older people are recognised as exhibiting frailty[7] characterised by unintentional weight loss, exhaustion, muscular weakness, slowed mobility and reduced physical activity. Frailty becomes increasingly likely with rising age and is predictive of disability, need for hospital care and death. In addition, older people are more likely to live with multiple long-term conditions.[8] The presence of multiple morbidities, which coexist but are not necessarily codependent, makes determination of outcome for an individual extremely difficult. Some of those outcomes – for example, future location of care – will cross the traditional domains of health and social care. As a result, many decisions about healthcare for older people can no longer be considered in isolation from the provision of social care.

Together with the development of complex systems of delivery, communication about health and social care is becoming ever more difficult. Care professionals are required to share information but may be constrained from doing so in ways that would otherwise give a more complete picture to the patient and his or her family.[9] Uncertainty about outcome is of increasing importance in assisting patients in making choices and yet communicating uncertainty without causing confusion is challenging. Physical and mental impairments may in addition hinder the normal dialogue between doctor and patient, thereby obstructing the usual consent process. At worst, this leads to a complete failure of the process, either because the patient is unable or unwilling to provide consent or because the doctor is unable or unwilling to seek consent. Sometimes the decision at hand seems too difficult or too overwhelming for the individual to make, and sometimes there is dispute about various aspects of the decision among the parties involved. The following case examples illustrate these problems.

CASE 3.1 **A patient unable to provide consent**

Dr Smith wishes to obtain a sample of blood from her patient Harry, who suf-ferers from dementia and is profoundly confused. He spends much of his day staring out of a window and he rarely talks. The doctor tries to explain her inten-tions to Harry, but he cries out loudly and pulls away when she lifts his arm and tries to insert the needle.

CASE 3.2 **A patient unwilling to provide consent**

Dr Smith wishes to obtain a sample of blood from her patient Sarah, who is awaiting surgery for a fractured neck of femur. The doctor tries to explain her intentions, but Sarah shrugs and says that at her time of life she does not want to be 'pulled about' and is much happier being left alone, 'whatever the consequences'.

CASE 3.3 **A doctor unable to seek consent**

Dr Smith wishes to obtain a sample of blood from her patient Pauline, who has severely impaired hearing and vision. The doctor tries to explain her intentions to Pauline, who smiles but does not otherwise respond. Dr Smith is left feeling uncertain as to how much has been understood.

CASE 3.4 **A doctor unwilling to seek consent**

Dr Smith wishes to obtain a sample of blood from her patient Michael, who has suffered a stroke and has expressive dysphasia. The doctor tries to explain her intentions to Michael, who attempts to respond but struggles to get the words out. Dr Smith listens to him struggling for a few minutes, but she is in a hurry and decides to proceed before Michael has finished trying to express himself. He becomes tearful during the procedure, and the doctor later worries about the correctness of her actions.

CASE 3.5 **An unremediable decision**

Albert has undergone a prolonged period of rehabilitation in a community unit supervised by Dr Smith. He has vascular dementia and has frequent episodes of urinary infection leading to delirium and falls. Despite limited recovery he con-tinues to be at high risk of falls when unsupervised, particularly at night when he wanders. He has had a home visit with the therapy team and could be sup-ported with social care visits, but he would be at high risk of self-neglect, falls and injury. He would be unsupervised at night. The team recommend moving him to a care home for safety. Albert wants to return to his own home where he feels he can 'be himself' in his 'own space' but he is unable to understand the risks entailed. His daughter contacts Dr Smith and tells her that she does not want Albert to return home and that he must move to a care home. She is not willing to support Albert in returning to his home.

CASE 3.6 Difficulties in determining ability to make a decision

Dr Smith is caring for Edna who has dementia and is in hospital following an episode of delirium causing a fall and self-neglect at home. When they discuss Edna's future care Edna indicates she wants to return to her own home to live with her husband, who in fact died 10 years ago. When reminded of this Edna becomes upset but seems able to understand that the care team have concerns about her continuing to live alone without support. She indicates that on reflection she wishes to move to a care home. Dr Smith attempts to explain that carers could be provided and she could be supported in her own home, at least for a while longer. Edna agrees to think about this, but a few hours later when Dr Smith repeats the earlier discussion, Edna has once more forgotten that her husband has died and she seems unable to make a choice about her future. Dr Smith is not clear in her own mind whether Edna is genuinely undecided what to do or whether she is unable to understand her circumstances well enough to make a choice.

By presenting a structured approach to the consent process, this chapter seeks to provide assistance in resolving dilemmas that are commonly encountered in delivering healthcare to older people. While it is tempting to resort to legal frameworks when deciding right from wrong, there are many situations where the law is unhelpful or even silent. A more pragmatic approach is to consider the moral basis of the consent process, and to work from first principles towards a solution that is consistent with the law, rather than dictated by it. Keeping sight of the values that underlie approaches to and execution of decisions is of immense importance to professionals and their patients alike.

THE BASIS OF CONSENT

Professional duties

It is helpful to look at the values that underlie the duties of health professionals. The various strands of professional practice on which the notion of consent is based are readily discernible in a variety of professional mandates. For example, in the Hippocratic oath[10] attention is drawn to the importance of acting only for a patient's benefit, and avoiding doing the patient harm:

I will prescribe regimen for the good of my patients according to my ability and judgement and never do harm to anyone ... In every house where I come I will enter only for the good of my patients, keeping myself far from all intentional ill-doing.

The General Medical Council, in setting out its guiding principles, has focused on the importance of patient-centred communication, partnership and respect, as follows.
➤ You must listen to patients, take account of their views, and respond honestly to their questions.
➤ You must give patients the information they want or need to know in a way they can understand. You should make sure that arrangements are made, wherever possible, to meet patients' language and communication needs
➤ You must be considerate to those close to the patient and be sensitive and responsive in giving them information and support.
➤ When you are on duty you must be readily accessible to patients and colleagues seeking information, advice or support.[11]

The moral basis of consent
Although specifically directed towards doctors, intuitively these declarations are more generally applicable. On closer inspection, three common themes emerge:
1. avoiding intentional harm
2. promoting benefit and well-being
3. respecting the wishes and desires of the individual.

Each of these themes relates to a particular moral principle (although this particular framework is not without criticism[12]), and it is helpful to consider each of them in turn.

Non-maleficence
This principle creates an obligation not to do intentional harm to others, and there are a number of ways of achieving this. Most obviously we should try not to do things that cause harm, but we may also be obliged to stop or prevent processes that are causing harm to an individual. It is helpful to decide what we mean by 'harm' in this situation. Although we ordinarily think of harm as meaning physical or psychological injury, there are other ways in which the interests of an individual may be damaged.

Returning to Dr Smith and her blood samples, we might conclude that Harry has been physically harmed when he cries out on being touched, but Michael's tearfulness also suggests harm, despite his showing no resistance to the procedure. This may be more than the pain of having blood taken, and may equally well relate to his thwarted attempts to express a view. In Sarah's case, the patient has expressed clearly that she does not want a blood test and that she is best left alone. Ignoring her wishes would both undermine her interests in being left alone and damage the trust that she maintains with her carers. Such action may thus harm the integrity of future decisions.

The cases of Albert and Edna are more difficult. Albert's risk of physical harm from falls and self-neglect must be balanced against the potential harms of overriding his express wishes to return to his own home. From the doctor's and relative's perspectives the tangible harms of injury and self-neglect are both anticipated and to some extent predictable, while the harms entailed in loss of home environment and potential for depersonalisation are more diffuse. Albert's cognitive impairment may make it more difficult for him to assimilate and assess the relative magnitudes of these harms, to balance them and to communicate his rationale for his choices. In Edna's case her cognitive disorder appears to prevent assimilation of the information that would help her to choose, but she also appears genuinely uncertain.

In situations such as these, understanding and weighing up direct, tangible harms is always going to be difficult, for the patient, for the patient's family and for care professionals. Where the patient genuinely has no prospect of doing this consistently, those who are left to make the decisions must give cognisance to the indirect, diffuse harms and weigh these as carefully as they would the direct harms. Failure to do so could represent a failure of the duty to maximise opportunity.

Beneficence

This principle requires us to act so as to contribute to the welfare of individuals and is closely allied to non-maleficence. We might choose to do this by actively providing benefit for a person, or by not restricting opportunities for benefit. Alternatively, we may choose to balance the benefits and drawbacks of a situation in order to arrive at the best outcome.

Dr Smith's cases provide some illustration of this principle. Her intention in obtaining the blood samples is presumably to derive information that will contribute to the welfare of her patients. By having open discussions with the patients, she has sought to avoid restricting their opportunities. If the patient has expressed a view, at least it can be taken into account. By balancing the benefits and drawbacks for her patient, the doctor may be better placed to arrive at a decision on how to proceed. Such a calculation would depend on factors such as the magnitude of benefit to be derived from doing the test, and the amount of harm done by overriding any objections that the patient might have.

Application of the beneficence principle is more difficult in the cases of Albert and Edna deciding where to live in future. For Albert the tangible benefit of moving to a care home derives from the reduction in risk of harm through injury and self-neglect. However, from the patient's perspective the benefits derive more from preservation of his sense of independence and self. The difficulty for professionals and his family relate to the calibration of these benefits against each other, given Albert's impaired ability to make decisions. On one reading of this scenario, his daughter attaches much greater benefit to protection from harm than does Albert himself. Is it right that Albert's assessment is devalued by his cognitive impairment? It is possible even to compare the relative value that attaches to different conceptions of benefit (avoidance of harm versus preservation of self and independence)?

If the principle professional duty lies in maximising opportunity for benefit, Dr Smith must try to ensure that her role is deployed in giving clarity and weight to Albert's personalised benefits. She must ensure that the balancing of benefits is fair and patient focused, rather than unbalanced by the more clearly articulated but, to Albert at least, less important benefits identified by professionals and family members.

Respect for autonomy

Respect for the wishes of an individual is perhaps at the root of morally robust consent. The concept of autonomy, although difficult to grasp, comprises elements of freedom from interference and capacity for action. In deciding whether to be influenced by an individual's views, it is useful to consider whether he or she is or can be autonomous. One view is that someone is autonomous if he or she:

➤ has plans free from interference by others
➤ has thought about these plans critically
➤ is free to carry out his or her plans.

Thinking about Dr Smith's patients, it could be argued that Harry's dementia prevents him from being autonomous. He does not appear to have the mental capacity to think about any plans. If he does have plans, his impairment is likely to constrain him in their execution. It could be argued that overriding his refusal does not conflict with the principle of respect for autonomy, since he is not autonomous. Sarah, on the other hand, clearly wants to be left alone, 'whatever the consequences': this seems to indicate that she has at least considered that there may be consequences to her refusing the test. Adherents to the principle of respect for autonomy would be unable to justify overriding her refusal, unless other grounds for questioning her autonomy could be found.

Where there is sufficient evidence that an individual is autonomous, it is difficult to justify proceeding in the face of a clear refusal. However, where the evidence to establish autonomy is lacking, decisions about an individual's autonomy can be difficult. In this situation it is useful to consider instead the notion of an *autonomous choice*.[13] What matters here is whether the individual has *actually* made a free decision about his or her care, rather than whether he or she is capable of being autonomous. It is the qualities of the decision that matter rather than the characteristics of the person making the decision. Dr Smith and her patients provide a useful illustration of this. Although Harry's dementia deprives him of autonomous status, he has nevertheless clearly indicated that he does not want a needle stuck in his arm. Whatever the reason for this response, it is a powerful demonstration that despite his dementia, he can still state a preference to be left alone.

Albert's case illustrates this point further still. He has expressed his will to return home and has given some reasons for making this choice. The difficulty here is that he may not be free to carry out his plan. His daughter does not support it and the professional team are reluctant because of their desire to reduce his tangible risks of harm. Nor does it appear that Albert has thought about his plans critically. For Edna the situation is even more difficult. She appears to have professional support in executing her plan and in the context of an isolated discussion appears able to think about her plans. The problem is that she fluctuates in her abilities to do this and the outcome of her choice is inconsistent.

In law, capacity assessment is generally thought of as a functional process relating to the individual's capabilities. However, the cases of Albert and Edna suggest that autonomy is not a binary state that is either present or absent. What is at issue for these patients is both the robustness and the quality of evidence in support of an assertion that the patient is autonomous. This requires a qualitative judgement to be made by those involved in supporting decisions as to whether a choice is the product of an individual capable of being autonomous or whether the choice itself is sufficient to evidence autonomy.

In assessing capacity to make decisions within a legal framework, Dr Smith will be faced with making this judgement. Her professional duty to respect autonomy therefore requires her to make a judgement about the relative quality of both the choice being expressed by her patient and the way in which her patient arrived at that choice. Dr Smith must be in a position to benchmark these aspects of the choice her patient is expressing against both the legal and the professional framework standards within which she is operating. This requires her to be fully aware of both her legal and her professional obligations, but, most important, it requires her to be focused on what her patient is communicating and what lies beneath that communication.

PROBLEMS WITH RESPECT FOR AUTONOMY

The difficulties highlighted for Dr Smith question whether there is an over-reliance on the principle of respect for autonomy. The principle suggests that while a patient retains autonomy we should respect his or her choices, whatever the outcome and so long as others are not harmed as a consequence. When autonomy is absent, the patient's views are no longer central to decision-making. In a way, this lets health workers off the hook. They need no longer worry about a patient who is choosing 'unwisely', because that choice does not demand respect. Instead, the views of others decide what should happen. The practice of allowing health workers to determine whether an individual is autonomous could effectively displace the balance of power in making a decision away from the patient. Strict adherence to the principle of respect for autonomy could paradoxically lead to higher levels of paternalism if health workers are reluctant to grant their patients' autonomous status.

The problem arises from the view that autonomy is either present or absent. The solution lies with willingness to permit 'partial autonomy' and to treat patients as people. The right to determine what should happen to you could therefore be granted on either ability to choose or preservation of self (personhood).

Partial autonomy

Even in a 'free' society there are rules that restrict action and choice, so that no adult is completely autonomous. It is simply unrealistic to require a patient to have full autonomy before respecting his or her choices. However, is a patient who is able to order and choose between his or her various desires (e.g. to eat, mobilise, or be free from pain) deserving of respect? Is a patient whose decisions are more based on emotion than risk calculation any less deserving of our respect? Arguably, only a patient who after close scrutiny exhibits no discernible process of choosing should be excluded from the consent process.

Personhood

Loss of this characteristic may indeed justify excluding the patient from a decision about his or her healthcare. However, most individuals without full autonomy will continue to be recognised as persons. The presence of actions that display purpose, awareness and intent together with a recognition of 'self' by external observers should prompt respect for preservation of personhood. Despite his dementia, Harry still presents himself as a person to his carers. Arguably, the doctor should respect his choice because he remains a person despite being unable to demonstrate that he is an autonomous individual. Albert clearly expresses a sense of self in arriving at his decision to return home, despite not being capable of assimilating other factors such as the magnitude of personal risk entailed.

THE LEGAL BASIS OF CONSENT

Consent in clinical practice may assume a variety of guises, from an explicit, fully informed dialogue to a tacit, implied authorisation. It is also important to remember that a significant aspect of the consent process is to provide choice for the patient, and that the outcome of that process may be either acceptance or refusal of an intervention. It is certainly not the purpose of the consent process to secure acceptance at all costs.

A further point to be noted is that the consent is an authorisation or refusal of an intervention offered to a particular individual, and unjustified attempts to exclude that individual from the process are likely to conflict with the principles of non-maleficence, beneficence and respect for autonomy. In other words, obtaining consent (or refusal) from any individual other than the one to whom the intervention directly relates must be clearly justified both morally and by applicable legal frameworks.

To ensure the validity of the consent process, it is widely agreed that a number of elements are essential:

1. capacity
2. information
3. voluntariness.

Capacity

The notions of capacity and autonomy are closely related, and it has been demonstrated that decisions about whether an individual is autonomous can be troublesome, particularly where evidence in favour of autonomy is lacking. In English law the Mental Capacity Act 2005[14] is underpinned by the following five key principles.

1. An adult is presumed to have capacity unless proven otherwise.
2. Individuals should be supported as far as possible to make their own decisions.
3. An unwise decision does not mean that an individual lacks capacity.
4. A decision made for someone lacking capacity must be made in that person's best interests.
5. Anything done for someone lacking capacity must be the option that least restricts his or her basic rights and freedoms.

For the purposes of the Act, a person lacks capacity in relation to a matter if at the material time he or she is unable to make a decision for him- or herself because of an impairment or disturbance in the functioning of the mind or brain. This means that a person lacks capacity if:

➤ the person has an impairment or disturbance that affects the way his or her mind or brain works, and
➤ the impairment or disturbance means that the person is unable to make a specific decision at the time it needs to be made.

For legal purposes, capacity is either present or absent, but a decision about the capacity of an individual will depend on the specific circumstances of the consent situation. For example, where an intervention carries little risk and great benefit to the individual, there may be little information for the individual to comprehend and process, and the decision may not be difficult to make. In this situation, a patient with significant impairment may nevertheless be judged to have capacity to make the decision. Where the risks and benefits of a procedure are more finely balanced, the complexity of information necessary to arrive at a decision may increase, so that even unimpaired patients may have difficulty reaching the standard of capacity required to make the decision.

Capacity can be assessed by any suitably trained health or social care professional and considers an individual's ability to understand the relevant information provided, retain the information and use it to make a decision. The individual must then have the ability to communicate his or her decision. If there is a temporary impairment of cognition (e.g. during a delirium), it must be considered whether a particular decision can wait.

Information

The information provided can influence decisions about capacity, but it can also influence the consent process in other ways. The notion of fully informed consent is particularly problematic. How much information does a patient actually require to make the decision? The patient may be at a distinct disadvantage if the professional decides to withhold certain facts. The reasons for doing so may be perfectly valid. For instance, if the information is considered harmful to the patient, or the professional simply does not know the facts.

In addition to problems of disclosure, consent may be obstructed by problems of understanding. The demonstration of understanding can be difficult and requires considerable experience. Dr Smith's discussion with Sarah illustrates the point well. She expresses the view that at her age she does not want to be treated, but this may be based on the mistaken belief that nothing can be done for older people with fractured hips. Although competent, she has misunderstood the purpose of the intervention because of a defect in the information she has been given. In the case of Edna the problem is more that of retaining key information, such as the death of her husband, although at the time of delivery she appears capable of understanding.

A useful approach to problems of information is to address the needs of the individual, and it is important to check with the patient that he or she has enough information to make a decision. Where understanding is in question, it may be prudent to wait (if the urgency for the intervention is not great) until understanding is sufficient. This may mean spending considerably more time than is usual in ensuring that information has been properly communicated and understood. There is no good substitute for repeated conversations over a period of time.

Voluntariness

Healthcare decisions should be free from undue influence, and here it is helpful to refer again to the principle of respect for autonomy. The patient may be influenced by the views of the health worker, while physical or cognitive impairments may also restrict freedom in making choices. It should also be remembered that patient freedom might be viewed in a positive sense of providing all available opportunities, or in a negative sense of not restricting opportunity.

Let us return to the case of Michael. His expressive dysphasia considerably limited his powers of expression, and in such situations it may be easier for the patient to nod an agreement than to try to explain his or her reasons for refusal of a procedure. Similar arguments could be mounted for Pauline, whose profound sensory impairments limit her freedom of expression and communication. In this sense, and for a variety of reasons, neither of these patients could be said to be truly free to make their own decisions.

Where a patient is either unwilling or unable to provide consent, it is helpful to consider whether the individual is free from adverse influence. Such influence may be either intrinsic as a consequence of his or her impairments, or extrinsic as a result of coercion by others. In the case of Albert, the strongly held view of his daughter that he should not return home could constitute undue influence. An effort should be made to address these issues and to reduce their impact on choices, thereby improving the validity of the consent process.

THE FORM OF CONSENT

When an intervention such as a surgical procedure is perceived to be of sufficient importance, the ritual of making the consent explicit may involve written documentation or a structured conversation with the patient. Where the intervention is more 'trivial', the patient's agreement may be assumed and the issue of consent then becomes tacit or implied. In the latter situation it is easy to forget about the need for consent altogether. It is important not to get complacent and to avoid slipping into assumptions that all decisions are made tacitly or are trivial.

Making the consent process explicit in all clinical encounters could rapidly undermine the smooth and efficient administration of healthcare, to the ultimate detriment of the patient. For example, it would be ludicrous to expect written documentation of agreement for each of the tasks entailed in day-to-day care. Nevertheless, the absence of explicit consent does not equate to the absence of need for consent, and it must be remembered that consent is an issue whenever a healthcare intervention is contemplated.

Of increasing concern for frail older people is the effect of complexity and risk surrounding particular types of decision. The cases of Albert and Edna illustrate this well. Where a significant change in circumstances, such as move to a care home, is contemplated following admission to hospital, considerable time may have to be invested in arriving at a robust decision. This can lead to delay in delivery or transfer of care, which while not intrinsically part of the healthcare decision must nevertheless be weighed in terms of the attendant benefits, harms and contribution to loss of respect for autonomy. At its worst the delay entailed in making a complex decision about future location of care can lead to the opportunity for choice being removed altogether, as an economically constrained health and social care system is increasingly incapable of accommodating a patient throughout this process.[15] This additional harm cannot be ignored by health and social care professionals, for reasons both pragmatic and moral, in the context of an expanding population of older people exhibiting frailty. For these reasons, consent for older people is as much an issue for health and social care commissioners and policymakers as it is for practitioners.

WHEN THERE IS NO VALID CONSENT

Despite the ubiquitous nature of consent, there will be many situations in the delivery of care to older people where there is simply no valid consent or refusal to be obtained. It will be clear that acceptance of this state of affairs should not be taken lightly, since due consideration must be given to factors that may be blighting the consent process. In addition, the moral validity of a consent process may be influenced by the values of health workers themselves, depending, for example, upon their particular conception of respect for autonomy or non-maleficence.

The Mental Capacity Act 2005 in England and Wales enables individuals to appoint an attorney with lasting powers to make decisions about welfare, property and affairs on their behalf should they lose capacity. However, uptake of these legal devices to aid decisions and advance care planning for individuals without capacity has been poor.[16] If there is no legally valid welfare representative or articulation of prior refusals of care, then decisions must be made in a person's best interests.

Best interests

The best interests process specifically does not apply where (1) a competent individual has already made an explicit advance refusal of the healthcare intervention being proposed, and (2) in some instances relating to research. All interested parties should meet to try to decide what the person would have wished had he or she had capacity to make his or her own decisions.

The Mental Capacity Act 2005 helpfully provides guidance to ensure that all relevant issues have been considered, as follows.

➤ Determining best interests cannot be simply based on age, appearance, condition or behaviour.
➤ All relevant circumstances should be considered.
➤ Every effort should be made to encourage and enable the person who lacks capacity to take part in the decision.
➤ If there is a chance that capacity will be regained, consider putting off the decision until this occurs.
➤ Particular caution must be applied to decisions about life-sustaining treatment, and in cases of dispute legal advice must be sought.
➤ The person's past and present wishes and feelings, beliefs and values should be taken into account.
➤ Intrinsic to the process is the careful weighing of benefits and harms related to the decision at hand.
➤ There is an obligation to ensure that the decision made is least restrictive to the individual to whom it relates.
➤ The views of others close to the individual should be considered.

As much background as possible about the person should be obtained, and any relatives or close contacts should be included in the process. If a person has no family or friends to advocate on his or her behalf, then an independent advocate should be arranged to support the decision-making process. The decision-making team must weigh the interests that an individual might have in receiving an intervention compared with those he or she might have in not receiving it. Such a calculation might involve weighing the pain and suffering likely to be caused against the possible benefits of having the procedure. This will in turn depend on the nature of the procedure.

For example, Dr Smith is likely to cause Harry great distress by persisting in taking blood, but the balance of interests in having the test will shift according to the reason for taking the blood. If the test is for a research project, the outcome of which is unlikely to benefit Harry, then it is unlikely to be in his best interests. However, if it is to cross-match blood for a much-needed transfusion, the balance of interests shifts the other way. Individual and professional values should not be allowed to influence unduly the decision-making process. For Albert this means that the views of his daughter, while being taken into account, must not be the sole determinant of the decision finally made.

CONSENT TO RESEARCH

The morality of the consent process with regard to research involving older people is essentially no different from that of other healthcare interventions. Nevertheless, the continued evolution of research ethics committees as 'gatekeepers' in the conduct of research involving vulnerable people has ensured that the consent process for research is generally more explicit and complete than in other aspects of clinical practice.[17]

An area of particular difficulty relates to research involving patients for whom there is no valid consent or refusal (e.g. those with severe dementia). Surrogate decisions in this context are more problematic, since the benefits to the patient may be less obvious, unknown or even non-existent. It is unlikely that interests will weigh strongly in favour of conducting the research. It is equally unlikely that a valid advance decision about care will have anticipated the nature of future research in sufficiently specific detail to permit authorisation.

Once again, strict adherence to the principle of respect for autonomy is problematic. As a result of excluding from research those patients who are unable to consent, both their condition and its treatment remain less well understood. Arguably this is just as morally unacceptable as engaging in experimentation on vulnerable adults without seeking their agreement. A way forward is to permit decisions by adults who have partial autonomy or who retain the characteristics of personhood. In practice, this might involve respecting the patient's sustained agreement to participate in research in the absence of obvious refusal. However, it is likely that research ethics committees will remain reluctant to authorise such an approach because of the potential for mistreatment.

KEY POINTS

- Freely given consent to healthcare is a moral and legal imperative.
- There has been increasing drive towards person-centred care and shared decision-making over the last decade, particularly for vulnerable adults.
- For older people, problems may arise because a patient is unwilling or unable to provide consent, or because the carer is unwilling or unable to seek consent.
- It is important to recognise when a decision is genuinely difficult and to allow adequate time to make decisions where possible.
- An understanding of the moral basis of consent will help to provide solutions to consent problems that are consistent with the law.
- The moral basis of consent is derived from the principles of non-maleficence, beneficence and respect for autonomy.
- Reliance on a narrow approach to respect for autonomy may lead to paternalism by excluding individuals who can still choose despite cognitive impairment.
- Respect for personhood and self is important in giving weight to decisions for people without capacity.
- A morally and legally valid consent requires the patient to be competent, informed and voluntary.
- Consent may be explicit or tacit, but it is relevant to all healthcare interventions.
- When an adult cannot provide valid consent, healthcare decisions may be justified on the basis of best interests or in line with valid advance decisions for care.

REFERENCES

1. Harris J. Consent and end of life decisions. *J Med Ethics*. 2003; **29**(1): 10–15.
2. Innes A, Macpherson S, McCabe L. *Promoting Person-Centred Care at the Front Line*. York: Joseph Rowntree Foundation; 2006.
3. O'Keeffe M, Hills A, Doyle M, *et al*. National Centre for Social Research; King's College London. *UK Study of Abuse and Neglect of Older People: prevalence survey report*. London: Comic Relief and Department of Health; 2007.
4. Coulter A. Do patients want a choice and does it work? *BMJ*. 2010; **341**: c4989.
5. Francis R. *Independent Inquiry into Care Provided by Mid Staffordshire NHS Foundation Trust January 2005–March 2009*. Vol. 375. London: TSO; 2010.
6. Neuberger J, Guthrie C, Aaronovitch D, *et al*. *More Care, Less Pathway: a review of the Liverpool Care Pathway*. London: Williams Lea; 2013.
7. Fulop T, Larbi A, Witkowski JM, *et al*. Aging, frailty and age-related diseases. *Biogerontology*. 2010; **11**(5): 547–63.
8. Barnett K, Mercer SW, Norbury M, *et al*. Epidemiology of multimorbidity and implications for health care, research, and medical education: a cross-sectional study. *Lancet*. 2012; **380**(9836): 37–43.
9. Shaw S, Rosen R, Rumbold B. *What is Integrated Care?* London: Nuffield Trust; 2011.
10. Cruess, Richard, and Sylvia Cruess. Updating the Hippocratic oath to include medicine's social contract. *Med Educ*. 2014; **48**(1): 95–100.
11. General Medical Council. *Good Medical Practice*. Manchester: GMC; 2013.
12. Lee MJ. The problem of 'thick in status, thin in content' in Beauchamp and Childress' principlism. *J Med Ethics*. 2010; **36**(9): 525–8.

13. Beauchamp TL, Childress JF. *Principles of Biomedical Ethics*. 6th ed. New York: Oxford University Press; 2008.
14. *Mental Capacity Act 2005*. London: Office of Public Sector Information. Available at: www.legislation.gov.uk/ukpga/2005/9/contents (accessed 24 March 2014).
15. Majeed MU, Williams DT, Pollock R, *et al*. Delay in discharge and its impact on unnecessary hospital bed occupancy. *BMC Health Serv Res*. 2012; **12**: 410.
16. Aw D, Hayhoe B, Smajdor A, *et al*. Advance care planning and the older patient. *QJM*. 2012; **105**(3): 225–30.
17. Chalmers D. Viewpoint: are the research ethics committees working in the best interests of participants in an increasingly globalized research environment? *J Intern Med*. 2011; **269**(4): 392–5.

CHAPTER 4

Decisions on life-sustaining therapy: nutrition and fluid

Martin J Vernon

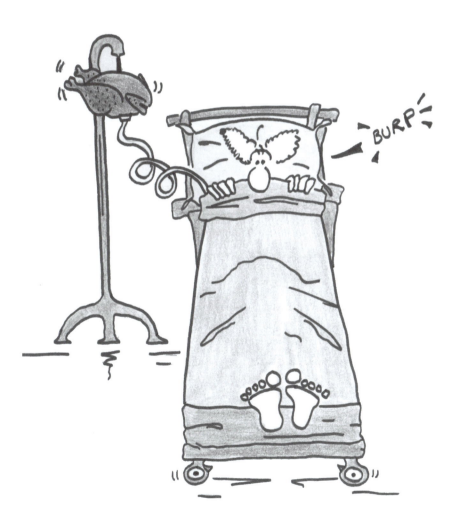

INTRODUCTION

The continued receipt of food and water is unarguably fundamental to life. If life is to be afforded value, then denying an individual these essential substrates seems morally indefensible. The terms starvation and dehydration appear to carry significant weight, particularly when associated with death as an outcome. Is this moral or emotional weight? Or both? What should you do when a person is nearing the end of his or her natural life? When that life is close to its inevitable end, does its intrinsic value change or even decrease? Does the imperative to sustain that life through the provision of food and water, by whatever means, become diminished? Is there a point at which there is no imperative to feed and hydrate? How and when can you make the judgement that food and water is no longer necessary?

The older population is expanding globally, and this is set to accelerate more so in less well economically developed countries.[1] While this is a marker of successful human ageing it means that in absolute terms more people than ever before are likely to achieve their natural life expectancy. Many of these people will exhibit frailty syndromes with poor physiological reserve, challenged nutritional status and, following acute illness, limited potential for recovery. The issues surrounding nutrition and hydration in the care of older people, particularly towards the end of their natural lives, will pose increasing challenge to health professionals and to those responsible for delivering a sustainable health and social care system.

There has long been media and political attention to the obvious link between healthcare delivery and the provision of nutrition and fluid.[2,3] While raising public awareness, there is nonetheless a danger of oversimplification and populism. In England in 2007, the Department of Health responded to the issue by producing an action plan[4] to improve nutritional care, which focused on older people. It highlighted the importance of issues such as screening, protected mealtimes and education of staff throughout healthcare settings. However, in 2011 the Care Quality Commission inspected 100 National Health Service (NHS) hospitals, focusing on their ability to meet required standards for dignity, nutrition and hydration in older people.[5] While 45 hospitals met the required standards the majority failed to satisfy the inspectors. The commission's report cited issues such as failing to assist patients with eating and prevention of meal completion by frequent interruptions.

Robert Francis QC[6] highlighted similar poor care in 2013 in his report of the Mid Staffordshire NHS Foundation Trust Public Inquiry. Francis[6] cited inadequate professional resourcing as a causative factor of inadequate treatment that at times could be characterised as abuse of vulnerable persons. He recommended that arrangements for providing food and drink to older people in hospital require implementation with 'constant review and monitoring'. It remains to be seen whether this will happen.

In the next 20 years the number of people in the UK aged over 85 will more than double and will account for 5% of the population.[7] Half of these people will have multiple long-term conditions. People with long-term conditions account for 70% of all inpatient bed days, 64% of outpatient appointments, 50% of general practitioner consultations and a significant portion of the total health and social care spend. Given that food poverty is increasingly recognised in developed countries[8] alongside rising economic poverty among older people,[9] nutrition is not just a health issue but also a macroeconomic and political issue of increasing magnitude and importance. In the UK alone malnutrition has been estimated to affect up to 3 million people, accounting for £13 billion of public expenditure.[10]

Older people are therefore at risk of malnutrition for a variety of reasons. The numbers of malnourished people in NHS hospitals in England has continued to rise dramatically: the estimated prevalence of malnutrition in general hospitals is at least 20%. Despite this, 70% of cases are undiagnosed and in up to 80% no action is taken during the hospital admission.[11] In one of very few UK hospital studies, up to 40% of acute admissions to elderly care wards were judged to be undernourished, with one in five severely so. In comparison, only one in 12 general medical and one in 100 general surgical admissions were severely undernourished.[12] The same study revealed that most of those who were undernourished on admission became more so during their hospital stay. Similar findings have been reported elsewhere.[13]

What remains unclear is the causal relationship between malnutrition and hospitalisation. Malnutrition is both a marker and a cause of poor health. How much hospitals contribute to worsening nutritional status and how much is simply physiological decompensation is unknown. Whatever the relationship, it does seem clear that healthcare systems are not skilled at either systematic recognition or treatment of malnutrition. It is little surprise that other studies have identified a relationship between malnutrition and increased mortality, rate of complications, length of stay and readmission rates.[14-16]

DECIDING HOW TO TREAT AN OLDER PERSON

When deciding whether or not to feed or hydrate an older patient who is, as a result of his or her condition, unable to take sufficient food and fluid orally, three main strands of argument commonly emerge.
1. Is there any clinical evidence that supports a particular course of action?
2. How technically feasible is it to pursue that course?
3. What are the guiding principles and values underlying those actions?

Clinical evidence

What is the evidence that clinical assistance with feeding an older patient will do some good? Conversely, is there evidence that feeding will do harm? Malnutrition affects many organ systems, leading to (among other things) impairments of central nervous, cardiorespiratory and immune function, cognition and tissue repair.[17] Patients who are already challenged by physiological ageing and by pathological changes in one or more of these systems are more likely to suffer the consequences of malnutrition, leading to increased healthcare costs, poor functional outcomes and death. The inference of this is that supplemental nutrition may reduce the impact of some or all of these effects, speeding recovery and reducing the length of hospital stay for patients following an acute illness. This notion has been confirmed in some studies of older patients undergoing rehabilitation.[18,19]

A 2011 Cochrane evidence review that focused on the effects of oral dietary supplementation in older patients concluded there was only limited evidence of benefit. While it is possible to produce a small gain in weight by using supplements, this did not translate to an overall survival benefit.[20] Similarly, a recent review concluded that there was insufficient evidence to recommend routine use of oral nutritional supplements in undernourished community-dwelling and institutionalised older people and those discharged from hospital.[21]

Following clinical practice changes in the use of percutaneous endoscopic gastrostomy (PEG) between the 1980s and 2000, this procedure was used increasingly for older patients with cerebrovascular disease. During this time, 30-day mortality rates reported in one UK study more than doubled to 19%.[22] In 2004 the UK National Confidential Enquiry into Patient Outcome and Death investigated PEG insertion for the purposes of administering food and fluid.[23] Of the procedures assessed, 95% were planned, with 82% being for patients aged over 70. The reported outcome of these procedures makes dismal reading: 43% died within a week and a further 26% died in the second week. A fifth (19%) of all procedures were considered to be futile from the outset. The report questioned the quality of information provided to patients and their relatives in agreeing to the procedure. In the United States, evidence that over 70% of hospitalised and 40% of nursing home patients died within 30 days of PEG led to a recommendation in 2000 that the procedure should be avoided altogether.[24]

Half of patients who have a non-fatal stroke will have difficulties in swallowing (dysphagia), of whom half will recover within 2 weeks, some will die and others will require long-term tube feeding. Optimal treatment of these patients remains unclear. An evidence review in 2012 suggested that starting tube feeding within 7 days of stroke onset may improve survival, but there were insufficient data to demonstrate that tube feeding improves overall mortality and functional outcomes following stroke.[25] At the onset of stroke there is at present no means to identify those patients likely to benefit from nutritional supplementation and those unlikely to benefit or those likely to suffer harm.

There are perhaps some benefits to clinically assisted nutrition, however. Nutritional supplementation following stroke may reduce the risk of pressure sore formation and similar evidence has been found following hip fracture, although supplementation does not also improve mortality. Again, however, there is as yet no means by which those likely to benefit can be easily identified.

In dementia the loss of normal physiological drivers of appetite due to changes in hypothalamic and limbic function, together with dysphagia in the latter stage, lead to emergence of malnutrition with involuntary weight loss.

Patients may simply lose interest in, or fail to recognise, food and fluid. This has led over the last 3 decades to increased use of tube feeding and hydration. In one US study of 186 835 nursing home residents with dementia, the prevalence of tube feeding was 34% yet there was no evidence of benefit in terms of prolonged survival, improved quality of life, nutritional status or risk of pressure sores developing.[26] There is also some evidence of harm from tube feeding through increased risk of developing pneumonia. In 2010 the Royal College of Physicians recommended careful hand-feeding of patients with dementia nearing the end of life and that PEG should not be used because the mortality is higher than without a feeding tube.[27]

There is evidence that supplementary feeding of malnourished people may in some circumstances cause harm. Re-feeding syndrome is caused by a potentially lethal shift in fluid and electrolytes, which results from hormonal and metabolic changes in turn caused by the rapid reintroduction of food after a period of established malnutrition. This rare but potentially survivable phenomenon is as yet poorly understood and emphasises the need to carefully identify patients at risk before proceeding to feeding, which must be then implemented with caution and close monitoring.[28]

At the end of life, whatever the cause, a person's desire for food may reduce. Often patients do not appear to experience hunger or thirst and attempting to eat normally can induce or worsen nausea and abdominal discomfort.[29] In a meta-analysis of 70 prospective, randomised, controlled trials involving cancer patients, there was no identified clinical benefit from providing nutritional support.[30] For those with cognitive impairment there is little evidence that thirst or hunger is perceived, and patients often refuse to be fed by their carers.[31] A dry mouth is a poor indicator of state of hydration and may be equally associated with medications or mouth-breathing. Mouth hygiene and withdrawal of unnecessary medication may be the only useful or, indeed, necessary interventions.

Therefore, when contemplating supplemental feeding and hydration, it is important first to consider the alternative options. For patients with advanced dementia who are experiencing swallowing difficulties, stopping anticholinergic medication, sedatives, neuroleptics or non-steroidal anti-inflammatory drugs may be sufficient to improve their nutritional intake. Any reversible illnesses such as infection or depression should be treated. Missing or ill-fitting dentures should be remedied. Mouth care should be provided. Other strategies include the education of care staff in how to safely feed patients at risk, the use of strong flavours and finger foods, or a change in the frequency and size of meals. With such measures, survival rates with or without nutritional and fluid supplementation may be no different.[32]

Technical feasibility

Where support of nutrition and/or hydration may be beneficial but oral feeding is impossible, what are the alternative means of accomplishing feeding? There is now a range of options at our disposal, including intravenous, subcutaneous, nasogastric, PEG, or radiographically inserted gastrostomy. However, in common with many other healthcare interventions, the availability of these techniques does not resolve the problem of whether it is right in the first place to employ this technology for a particular patient.

Guiding principles and values

Clarifying the clinical evidence, together with an understanding of what is possible, will focus the decision-making process. Although helpful, this approach alone may not yield a morally robust solution to a clinical dilemma. Where there is no evidence of benefit from an intervention, or there is evidence that it might do great harm, there may be little debate. Often, however, the evidence supports several courses of action to which there are no particular technical barriers. A decision must then be made as to the right course of action in each individual situation.

Two morally important questions commonly arise:
1. Should we feed (and/or hydrate) this person?
2. Should we stop feeding (and/or hydrating) this person?

The remainder of this chapter seeks to develop a framework for addressing these questions, and assumes that there is at least some clinical evidence in favour of the courses of action available, and that such actions are at least technically possible. In practice, nutrition and hydration are often provided together. However, current practice has also evolved around the use of a variety of techniques such as careful hand-feeding (where accepted) together with the use of intravenous or subcutaneous fluids. Some will view the mechanism of delivery as of no moral consequence and may view the provision of nutrition and hydration, whether orally, by tube or by drip, as part of the basic care of that person.

MEDICAL TREATMENT OR BASIC CARE?

In developing a morally robust solution to the dilemma of whether or not to feed an older patient, it is necessary to consider first whether nutritional support constitutes medical treatment or basic humane care. Those who support the view that it is medical treatment have invoked the moral imperatives driving good professional practice to decide on the appropriateness of proposed treatment.[33,34] Those who adhere to the view that food is a basic necessity of life, irrespective of how it is given, have developed arguments along more humanitarian lines, free from the encumbrances of professional codes of practice.

It is of note that the procedural nature of supplemental nutrition and hydration does seem to impact on its categorisation, and therefore too on the moral arguments that surround its application. Consider the clinical scenario outlined in Case 4.1.

CASE 4.1

Jodie has been admitted to hospital with pneumonia. At the time of admission, she is judged to be malnourished. She is given 'three square meals' of hospital food per day but continues to lose weight. She is reviewed by a dietician, who recommends supplementation and gives her cartons of liquid nutrients, which she enjoys drinking. One week after admission Jodie suffers a stroke and is unable to swallow. Nasogastric feeding is commenced and she makes good progress with rehabilitation. Unfortunately, 1 month later she is diagnosed with a carcinoma of the large bowel, which is threatening to obstruct. The surgical team is prepared to operate but first requests intravenous feeding to optimise her chances of recovery from the surgery.

At what point does the nutritional support that Jodie requires constitute medical therapy? 'Three square meals' does not appear to constitute medical therapy, since no specific procedure is involved and she is free to eat normally. The UK General Medical Council does not consider providing assistance to people who need help to eat or drink (e.g. by spoon-feeding) as a 'clinically assisted' procedure.

At first glance, it would appear that Jodie's meals assume the moral status of a basic necessity of life. Nevertheless, there is an alternative view. She is now in a clinical environment, which is by its nature therapeutic. It is not only the antibiotics she receives for her pneumonia that will help to restore her health but also the attentions and care of a full multidisciplinary team including nurses, therapists, dietician and doctors. The food she is receiving is part of this therapeutic process, and as such is subject to the same level of supervision and monitoring as other unarguably clinical therapeutic aspects of her care.

Further support for this view arises when it becomes necessary for a nurse or other skilled professional to supervise feeding, perhaps because the patient is at risk of aspiration. Although the patient may be consuming normal food, the process of eating can be achieved safely only with skilled intervention. Similar arguments could be presented for the liquid nutrition and hydration that Jodie is given. Such drinks are readily available outside the medical environment and could simply be viewed as food. Alternatively, they could assume the status of a treatment by assisting the management of her medical conditions, which have been worsened as a result of malnutrition and/or dehydration. This view is reinforced by the practice of *prescribing* these drinks, often on the advice of a dietician.

Nasogastric and intravenous feeding appear at first glance to be more in the realm of clinical treatment. They are invasive, require expertise to accomplish effectively and are provided in a clinical environment (at least at the outset). Are the technical aspects of the intervention simply confusing us? One could take the view that the intended outcome is simply to provide the patient with the food he or she requires in order to continue living. The medical equipment associated with feeding by these routes is necessary but morally irrelevant.

In the legal case of Anthony Bland, a man in a persistent vegetative state who was kept alive by nasogastric feeding, the Official Solicitor argued that clinically assisted nutrition and hydration was distinct from medical treatment: it was a basic necessity of life, without which he would die.[35] It was contended that doctors had a continuing duty to provide food and hydration to the patient, and that to discontinue them constituted manslaughter or even murder. In short, this would be a wilful neglect of basic human need. In response, the House of Lords took the view that the food and fluid given to Mr Bland was part of a treatment regimen. It was the way food and hydration was being given rather than what was administered that was of importance. The Lords concluded that the continuance of life for Anthony Bland was dependent on a comprehensive clinical regimen, of which nutritional support was an inseparable part. The appropriateness of continued feeding was judged on the basis that it was clinical treatment, not basic care. As such it might be withdrawn or withheld like any life-prolonging treatment, where commencing or continuing it was not in the patient's best interests.

This leads to the conclusion that the mechanism of providing nutrition and hydration is the critical factor in deciding whether it is legally permissible to stop treatment. One must conclude from this that the mechanism and setting of feeding and hydration interventions determines their legal status (in England at least). Interestingly, it does not appear to directly settle the moral worth of the interventions. Someone who does not regard the mechanism of food and fluid administration as having intrinsic value, but rather the food and fluid itself, might readily disagree with a decision to stop administering them.

NUTRITION AS MEDICAL TREATMENT

If nutrition is to be afforded the legal status of clinical treatment, the process of making decisions surrounding its use becomes clinically oriented, similar to when deciding the appropriateness of antibiotic therapy or surgery, for example. In this situation it becomes necessary to consider the expected outcomes of treatment and the wishes of the patient concerned.

Expected outcomes of treatment

Before commencing a treatment regimen, it is usual to consider the outcomes one is trying to achieve. Provision and consumption of nutrition and hydration has an impact on at least five outcomes:
1. prolonging life
2. creating health
3. preventing disease
4. relief of symptoms
5. opportunity for socialisation.

Before considering the moral significance of these outcomes, it is important to decide whether or not they can be achieved. This requires consideration of two further factors:

1. Could nutrition and/or hydration achieve the expected outcomes for any patient?
2. Could nutrition and/or hydration achieve the expected outcomes for this particular patient?

In other words, is there generalisable evidence to support the view that the proposed course of action works for this type of circumstance? Does that evidence apply in this particular circumstance, having taken all relevant information into account? It is not always easy to provide answers to these questions. As outlined earlier, there is little evidence in support of the hypothesis that nutrition achieves the outcomes of recovery to independence, or avoidance of harm through further illness or death for older people with progressive physiological failure towards the end of life. Health workers may have to draw on their own experiences and exercise judgement. The absence of robust clinical evidence or scientific data does not necessarily invalidate the subjective conclusions of a team of experienced professionals. However, it is important to ensure that subjective opinion is recognised as such and not permitted to assume the status of dogma. In other words, professional opinion can weigh in the decision process but it should not dominate it exclusively. Judgement of opinions and evidence, if that is what is required to make the decision, involves weighing of all relevant information, not just that of professionals.

Therefore, it is important that effort is made to assess the best available evidence, and that the effect of values of individuals in assessing the weight of such evidence is made explicit. The latter situation may occur when individuals are selective in articulating the evidence while influencing the final decision. This filtering process may come about through ignorance, but it may also be subject to the professional or personal values of those individuals. This is not to say that individual judgement has no role but simply that it should be exercised explicitly. Team awareness of the values in play is critically important to ensure that a balanced final decision is reached. Of even greater importance is team awareness of evidence filtering when communicating with the patient or his or her family, whether through the exercise of individual judgement, ignorance or as a result of value systems, declared or hidden. Failure to fully appreciate the impact of value systems that underpin a decision is likely to lead to poor communication with a patient and his or her family, thus undermining the quality of the decision made. It will also erode trust in the clinical team.

The second question involves assessment of the prognosis, a process that is also imprecise and subjective. This was highlighted in the UK 2013 Neuberger review of the Liverpool Care Pathway of the Dying.[36] Consider the scenario in Case 4.2, for example.

CASE 4.2

Albert is unable to safely swallow following a stroke. The stroke unit assesses him as having a 'reasonable' prognosis for good outcome. His doctor is aware of research evidence suggesting a benefit from the early use of PEG feeding following such a stroke. A request is made to the endoscopy service, but the endoscopist refuses on the basis that although the procedure is reasonably safe, the quoted evidence is of low quality. He also remarks that Albert's prognosis for functional recovery and anticipated future quality of life is 'appalling', and that he would not want a PEG tube for any relative of his following a stroke.

In this case the endoscopist is choosing to ignore evidence that the PEG tube might help Albert, in the absence of any clear evidence that it would definitely harm him. He is also introducing imprecise estimates of prognosis. Such views appear to be driven by the values of the endoscopist, who is opposed to PEG feeding for stroke patients in general. Judgement about quality of life, which cannot be measured in any meaningful way, appears to be driven by his personal values. Failure to remain objective while assembling evidence of benefit or harm will confuse discussion of the values attached to various clinical outcomes. Worse, the weighing in of personal values by a professional, that arguably have no legitimate place in the discussion, could lead to an unbalanced and unfair decision not to treat the patient. This is arguably a failure of professional duty to the patient.

The remedy in this situation would be for the endoscopist to declare that his personal values are influencing his judgement and are in conflict with his colleagues. On the grounds of conscientious objection he should pass the decision to a colleague who is better prepared to deploy only his or her professional value set in contributing to the outcome of the decision process. Even though the decision outcome may be the same, the process of making the decision will be more morally robust.

Having taken care to assemble the best evidence uncontaminated by personal values (unless overtly declared), and to make the best estimate of prognosis, the clinical team must attempt to determine the likelihood of achieving various outcomes. In practice, outcomes will be achieved to a greater or lesser degree, and it is necessary to estimate where the clinical intervention lies on the spectrum between success and failure. It is particularly important for the clinical team to declare if they simply do not know what the outcome will be, based on their assessment of the circumstances and evidence at hand. It is unreasonable to expect anyone, including clinicians, to offer absolute certainty about a particular outcome. While allowing clinical uncertainty may be unsettling for a patient or his or her family, it may also allow those involved to set aside the clinical issues and concentrate instead on what is possible and what value should be attached to various possible outcomes.

Deciding upon the relative value of outcomes is a process that will be influenced both by the circumstances of the patient and by the professional values of those involved in making the decision. If survival is to be valued above all else, then an intervention which has any impact on improving survival will be favoured, even at the expense of unwanted symptoms, side effects or compromise to other aspects of the person's health. Alternatively, those who value quality of life most highly may be prepared to accept an intervention that relieves symptoms but at the expense of reduced life expectancy.

There are several benefits of this approach. First, it enables the process of making decisions to be explicit and provides an opportunity to separate out the practical elements of a decision (will the treatment deliver given outcomes?) from the moral elements (which outcomes are most valued in this case?). Second, all individuals involved in the decision are permitted to reach a view separately at first, and then together as a group. Where conflict arises, it may be possible to address the problem by making explicit the values attached by individuals to the various treatment outcomes. Third, although the process requires assessment and ordering of the moral worth of various outcomes (a teleological or outcome-based approach), it also permits a rule-based (deontological) approach, should an individual choose to value one particular outcome (such as the preservation of life, or prevention of harm) above all else.

The wishes of the patient

If clinical support of food and fluid intake is to be regarded as medical treatment, then as with any other treatment it is necessary to seek the agreement of that individual before proceeding. Older people with frailty for whom such support is contemplated are often unable to participate fully in making decisions about their care because of their illness, and difficulties will arise when their wishes are not clear.

Approaches to this situation are outlined in Chapter 3, 'Informed consent', and the elements of the process are summarised as follows.

➤ Valid consent to treatment requires that the person has capacity, he or she is informed and the consent it is voluntary.

➤ To have capacity to decide about a treatment a person should, despite impairment of brain and mind function, be able to take in and retain information about the proposed treatment, balance the risks and benefits in his or her own mind, and arrive at and communicate his or her choice.

➤ If a person lacks capacity for a given decision and cannot participate, others must decide in a way that is morally and legally justifiable, ensuring that the outcome of that process is in his or her interests.

Surrogate decision-making about clinical support of nutrition and hydration is not without problems. In a follow-up study of individuals who decided to accept tube feeding for their elderly relative without capacity, two-thirds were satisfied with their decision and four-fifths would do the same again.[37] Even so, almost one-third of relatives in retrospect regret their decision.[38] Evidence that families are ill-informed about life-sustaining treatments suggests, however, that surrogates will require considerable education before being able to contribute meaningfully to a decision.[39]

One way to facilitate best interests decisions or make decisions in advance of loss of capacity is to engage older people in discussions about nutritional support in advance of their requiring it. In one large study, one-third of competent older individuals in nursing homes would elect to have a feeding tube in the event that they suffered 'brain damage' and were unable to eat.[40] A potentially useful approach to this is to identify and engage those most at risk early – for example, people with multiple long-term conditions, a frailty syndrome or early cognitive failure. This is of particular importance in those likely to require clinically assisted nutrition and/or hydration, such as patients with dementia or progressive neurodegenerative disease. At present such discussions are not commonplace but they appear acceptable to older people, they can be presented in an easily comprehensible format (e.g. using vignettes) and they do not provoke anxiety.[41] Given evidence that for those involved considerable education is required about proposed interventions, it is likely that advance care planning decisions may present problems with practicability.[42]

An advance decision or properly appointed welfare attorney may at best provide the information about what a patient now lacking capacity would have wished in these circumstances. If none is available, family members may still of course provide vital information on cultural, religious and personal beliefs and values that may affect the decision on whether to feed an individual artificially.

NUTRITION AS BASIC CARE

If nutritional support assumes the status of basic care, decisions about its use are often driven by beliefs, which surpass those employed in making a clinical treatment decision. In particular, it is the values attached to continued comfort, well-being and ultimately life that enable the correct course of action to be decided upon.

A framework that adheres to these values is set out in the ancient Jewish ethico-legal system known as *Halacha*.[43] In this system, the preservation of life takes precedence over virtually all other considerations. This stems from the belief that God has made man in his own image and in addition has given him the gift of life to be held in trust. Honouring and preserving this life is both a duty and a means of honouring God. Quality-of-life issues are of lesser importance, and only those measures that cause severe pain and suffering are to be avoided, specifically when a patient is moribund or death is imminent. In general, however, nutritional support, by whatever means, should not be refused or withdrawn, since to do so would hasten the patient's death.

Others who take a more moderate approach might view clinically assisted nutrition and hydration as 'extraordinary' treatment that might be refused in situations where the person is irreversibly and terminally ill. For example, patients with advanced dementia who have impaired swallowing may be considered terminally ill, given a median survival of only 6 months. Other moral frameworks have also employed the distinction between 'ordinary' and 'extraordinary' care in deciding about life-sustaining treatment. Care is extraordinary and therefore not obligatory if it involves great cost, pain or burden to the patient or to others, without reasonable chances of success.[44] Here the argument hinges on what you consider a successful outcome. If it is purely the maintenance of life, then life-sustaining care may be classed as ordinary. If success means more than this, perhaps the restoration of full health, then painful or costly care that does not achieve this outcome is considered extraordinary.

Opponents of this approach take the view that what is costly, painful or otherwise burdensome today might be cheap and trouble-free in the future. Indeed, the relative ease with which clinically assisted nutrition and hydration can now be provided has arguably led to its becoming 'ordinary' care, whereas 3 decades ago it might have been considered 'extraordinary'. Others might argue that because the expected outcomes of care determine its moral status, it is not the care that requires evaluation but, rather, its end points. According to this view it is less important to distinguish medical therapy from basic care, and more important to decide upon the value of the possible outcomes.

The most extreme *Halachic* view might override the values of the patient, perhaps on the grounds that no individual has the right to refuse that which gives life. Others would consider refusal only on the basis that it would prolong suffering and that otherwise every second of life is infinitely precious. In general, however, classifying nutrition as basic care removes some of the barriers to making decisions that might otherwise encumber patients and their family when attempting to participate in a strictly clinical decision. The complexity of making clinical decisions arguably makes it a less accessible process, whereas decisions based on values may be more accessible, balanced and fair to all participants.

SHOULD WE FEED/HYDRATE THIS PERSON WHO IS UNABLE TO MAKE THE DECISION?

In the absence of clear guiding evidence in support of commencing clinically assisted feeding and hydration, an ethical framework can be of help in supporting balanced and robust decisions. The framework proposed here (*see* Table 4.1) is not comprehensive. However, it may be used to give structure to the complex process of evaluating a particular case where a patient cannot participate because of lack of capacity. It allows all interested parties to be involved.

As with all morally important decisions, the expected outcome should be reviewed regularly to ensure that both the circumstances and the values on which the decision was based have not altered significantly over time. Where the decision was not to feed and/or hydrate, this will involve rehearsing once more the arguments already outlined. Once the decision has been taken to feed and/or hydrate a patient, there are a number of additional factors to be addressed prior to discontinuing feeding.

TABLE 4.1 An aid to decisions when considering the provision of clinically assisted nutrition and hydration to an older person unable to participate in the decision

Step	Understanding and awareness	Consideration and action

1	1. Are the reasons for this situation fully understood and all reversible factors treated?
	2. If not, is further action appropriate?
	3. What are the expected outcomes of care?
	  • Prolonging life
	  • Creating health
	  • Preventing further deterioration
	  • Relief of symptoms
	  • Opportunity for socialisation
	  • Are there others?
		1. Arrange a meeting with family, carers and members of the multidisciplinary team to discuss the following.
		  • Are the expected outcomes reasonable?
		  • Are there others not yet considered?
		  • What is the likelihood of success?
		  • What is the timescale for review of success in achieving outcomes and plans?
		2. Explore understanding about clinical circumstances and likely prognosis
		3. Consider the patient's prior wishes, values and beliefs
		4. Consider advocacy for the patient
		5. Make a clear decision about the use of clinically assisted nutrition and/or hydration

2a	1. Decision to provide clinically assisted nutrition and hydration 2. Decision not to provide clinically assisted nutrition and/or hydration	1. Agree deliverable outcomes for the treatment planned 2. Set a clear timescale for formal review of outcomes with family and multidisciplinary team members 3. Continual reassessment of condition mindful of agreed outcomes 4. Continual care to provide comfort and dignity 5. Regular communication with patient (where possible), family and team members 6. Continue to offer regular (during waking hours) hand-feeding and hydration as tolerated and accepted by the patient
2b	Unable to reach a decision	1. Seek second clinical opinion(s) focused on the considerations at Step 1 2. Ensure advocacy for key non-professional participants and the patient 3. Continue to offer regular (during waking hours) hand-feeding and hydration as tolerated and accepted by the patient 4. Consider the need for a formal legal declaration
3	Change of circumstances	Go back to Step 1

SHOULD WE STOP FEEDING/HYDRATING THIS PERSON WHO IS UNABLE TO MAKE THE DECISION?

Discussions about stopping food and/or fluids will occur when it is apparent that continuing to feed and/or hydrate is not the correct course of action. In practice, this may occur for one of two reasons:

1. circumstances have changed
2. values of those involved have changed.

Circumstances have changed

Where expected outcomes of care can be delivered without clinically assisted nutrition and/or hydration, perhaps because of improved patient prognosis, stopping will not be problematic. Examples include recovery of swallowing following a stroke, or restoration of consciousness following delirium.

CASE 4.3

Peter was admitted to hospital following a stroke 3 months ago. Because of swallowing difficulties, a PEG tube was inserted for feeding purposes. Despite comprehensive attempts at rehabilitation, Peter has made no progress and 1 week ago he suffered a second stroke, which has left him unconscious but otherwise clinically stable.

Difficulties are more likely to arise when the passage of time creates a clearer understanding of patient prognosis, leading to a change in the expected outcomes of care. This may occur when the patient deteriorates or fails to show any signs of improvement. Cases 4.3 and 4.4 illustrate these problems.

CASE 4.4

Cathy has a learning disability and was living in a residential home prior to admission. One month ago she developed septicaemia following a perforation of her colon. Following surgery to remove part of her large bowel, intravenous feeding was commenced to correct malnutrition and facilitate recovery. Despite attempts at rehabilitation, she has remained fully dependent on nursing care.

In the case of Peter, the expected outcomes of feeding included maintenance of life and good functional outcome from his stroke. Recent events indicate that the latter outcome is unlikely to be met, and discussion must now centre on the value attached to his continued living, together with any new outcomes such as relief of distressing symptoms. Meanwhile, Cathy is unlikely to achieve functional independence, although she shows no signs of further deterioration. Here the expected outcomes of care must alter. Rather than restoring functional independence, feeding is only likely to maintain present stability.

Discussion of the appropriateness of continued feeding must therefore involve evaluation of these new or reprioritised aims of treatment. While discussion here may focus on conversion to a less sophisticated means of feeding (such as PEG), it is nevertheless opportune to examine the values that underlie all forms of feeding rather than dwelling simply on its delivery mechanism. In practice, it is all too easy to ignore the wider purpose of treatment and settle decisions purely on narrow clinical grounds.

Values of those involved have changed

Having gained experience of the effects of feeding over a period of time, those involved in the decision to feed may choose to alter or reprioritise the values they originally attached to expected outcomes. For instance, the original decision may have been based on an overwhelming desire to maintain continued life, which has subsequently given way to the more valued outcome of relieving distress. This is illustrated by Case 4.5.

CASE 4.5

Joyce was left with speech and swallowing difficulties following evacuation of a subdural haematoma 2 months ago. After discussion with her daughter and in her best interests, it was decided to insert a PEG tube to facilitate feeding. Despite attempted rehabilitation, Joyce has made no progress and remains dependent for all nursing care. She has acquired pressure sores and she grimaces in pain when moved. Her daughter now feels that the need to preserve life does not justify Joyce's continued suffering.

When professionals and family have reached a decision together, a sustained change in the value attached to key outcomes by one party should prompt re-evaluation of the decision by all participants to the decision. This will again ensure that the basis of any new decision is explicit and based on clear expected outcomes of care. For example, the views of Joyce's daughter may alter if she is reassured that her mother's pain can be adequately controlled and that continued feeding may help her pressure sores.

Particular difficulties may arise when the values of the patient become altered by the passage of time – for instance, when a patient no longer wants nutritional support. Here it is helpful to retrace the decision-making process with the patient to clarify the basis of his or her new decision and to evaluate his or her competence to do so. In certain circumstances, legal clarification may be required. Case 4.6 illustrates this point.

CASE 4.6

June has suffered from Parkinson's disease for 8 years and has become severely malnourished. Three months ago she consented to have a nasogastric tube inserted to facilitate feeding. Despite adequate feeding, she has remained fully dependent and is awaiting admission to a nursing home. She has now decided that she does not wish to live in this condition and has made a refusal of further feeding via the tube.

Given that unconsented touching may constitute battery or assault, the legal implications of June's refusal for her carers are significant. Evaluating her decision may clarify whether she has the capacity to refuse feeding and may elucidate the values on which she bases her refusal. This will help her carers to decide on what basis they must either respect her wishes or override her refusal. If June has capacity and her decision is otherwise legally valid then her wishes must be respected, even if malnutrition ultimately results in her death.

KILLING OR LETTING DIE?

No decision about nutritional support will be free from the elements of this debate, which centres on the moral equivalence of acts (that constitute killing) and omissions (that result in death). Consider the scenario outlined in Case 4.7.

CASE 4.7

Jeremy suffered a stroke 1 year ago, which left him unable to swallow, and he had a PEG tube inserted. He now states that he wishes to die and requests that the tube be removed. This would require an endoscopic procedure, which the endoscopist refuses to undertake, on the grounds that her actions would ultimately lead to Jeremy's death. Instead, she recommends that the tube be left in place but not be used. Jeremy's nurse argues that this has the same effect and that he does not wish to stand by and watch his patient die by his omission.

The endoscopist believes that an action that leads to Jeremy's death has more moral weight than an omission that leads to the same outcome. She could argue that removing the tube causes Jeremy's death, and that she is therefore killing him by agreeing to his request. She could also argue that she is assisting in Jeremy's suicide or even that her actions constitute active voluntary euthanasia. The nurse, on the other hand, does not draw a distinction between an act or an omission, on the basis that the outcome is the same. His argument might focus on whether or not it is right for Jeremy to die, not on the means by which this outcome could be achieved.

One could argue that without the PEG tube, Jeremy's death would be inevitable, and the tube is merely a barrier to events for which his carers are not responsible. Tube removal does not constitute killing him; it is simply allowing him to continue his journey towards death. Others might argue that we are obliged to remove the tube out of respect for Jeremy's autonomous choice. In this case his death may be foreseen, but it is not an intended effect of our actions, simply a side effect.

Alternatively, you could argue that we have a duty of care to Jeremy, which includes providing effective barriers to his death. If we do not prevent his death, then we might also decide not to prevent the deaths of others. This might place us on a 'slippery slope' towards withholding treatment for all patients who are dying. Furthermore, as carers we have a duty to care, but not to undertake activities that compromise our own moral and professional standards. We are not obliged to do something to Jeremy that might lead directly to his death, even if he demands it.

There is no right or wrong solution to this dilemma, but it is important that those involved in such difficult decisions are individually comfortable with the outcome. There is no substitute to working through the arguments, guided by the framework outlined previously. Not only will this lead to a morally explicit decision but also this will facilitate discussion and progress in those difficult cases where legal clarification is the only way forward.

THE LAW

In English law, the majority of cases dealing specifically with nutrition have centred on the tube feeding of individuals without their consent, or the withdrawal of tube feeding from individuals unable to express their views. Some of the key issues are summarised as follows.

➤ Food is legally identified by its chemical composition, not by its form of administration.
➤ Liquid food does not therefore constitute medicine.
➤ Clinically assisted nutrition and/or hydration forms part of a regimen that amounts to medical treatment.
➤ Medical treatment generally may not be administered to a competent adult without his or her consent.
➤ In the case of adults without capacity to decide, clinically assisted feeding and/or hydration decisions should follow their best interests.
➤ Assessment of best interests usually includes discussion with family members and must include balancing of burdens and benefits, taking care to pursue the option that is least restrictive to the individual.
➤ There is no obligation to give treatment that is futile or excessively burdensome.
➤ The law regards withholding or withdrawing treatment as an 'omission', not an 'act'.
➤ When contemplating forced feeding or withdrawal, seek legal clarification.

KEY POINTS

- A decision to clinically assist with feeding and/or hydrating an older person requires consideration of the benefits, feasibility and morality of the proposed procedure.
- The expected outcomes of providing clinical assistance to nutrition and hydration should be explicit from the outset, be subject to continual review and be evaluated by estimating the ongoing likelihood of success.
- The wishes and values of the patient must be considered, either contemporaneously or in the form of advance statements.
- For patients who are unable to make decisions, a morally robust decision about clinical assistance with nutrition and hydration must be made after wide consultation with other clinicians and family members.
- Decisions to commence clinically assisted nutrition and hydration must be reviewed in the light of changing circumstances or the values of those making the decision.
- Decisions to stop or to impose clinically assisted feeding and hydration create complex moral problems that may require legal clarification.

REFERENCES

1. Population Reference Bureau. World population highlights: key findings from PBR's 2010 world population data sheet. *Population Bulletin.* 2010: **65**(2). Available at: www.prb.org.pdf1065highlights.pdf (accessed 24 March 2014).
2. Quill TE. Terri Schiavo: a tragedy compounded. *N Engl J Med.* 2005; **352**(16): 1630–3.
3. Racine E, Amaram R, Seidler M, *et al.* Media coverage of the persistent vegetative state and end-of-life decision-making. *Neurology.* 2008; **71**(13): 1027–32.
4. Department of Health. *Improving Nutritional Care: a joint action plan from the Department of Health and Nutrition Summit Stakeholders.* London: DH; 2007.
5. Care Quality Commission. *The State of Health Care and Adult Social Care in England in 2011/12.* Vol. 763. London: TSO; 2012.
6. Francis R. *Independent Inquiry into Care Provided by Mid Staffordshire NHS Foundation Trust January 2005–March 2009.* Vol. 375. London: TSO; 2010.
7. Donnelly G, Wentworth L, Vernon MJ. Nutrition, older people and the end of life. *Clin Med.* 2013; **13**(Suppl. 6): S9–14.
8. Dowler EA, O'Connor D. Rights-based approaches to addressing food poverty and food insecurity in Ireland and UK. *Soc Sci Med.* 2012; **74**(1): 44–51.
9. Donini LM, Scardella P, Piombo L, *et al.* Malnutrition in elderly: social and economic determinants. *J Nutr Health Aging.* 2013; **17**(1): 9–15.
10. Guest JF, Panca M, Baeyens JP, *et al.* Health economic impact of managing patients following a community-based diagnosis of malnutrition in the UK. *Clin Nutr.* 2011; **30**(4): 422–9.
11. Lean M, Wiseman M. Malnutrition in hospitals. *BMJ.* 2008; **336**(7639): 290.
12. McWhirter JP, Pennington CR. Incidence and recognition of malnutrition in hospital. *BMJ.* 1994; **308**(6934): 945–8.
13. Burgos R, Sarto B, Elío I, *et al.* Prevalence of malnutrition and its etiological factors in hospitals. *Nutr Hosp.* 2012; **27**(2): 469–76.

14. Incalzi RA, Capparella O, Gemma A, *et al.* Inadequate caloric intake: a risk factor for mortality of geriatric patients in the acute care hospital. *Age Ageing.* 1998; **27**: 303–10.

15. Kagansky N, Berner Y, Koren-Morag N, *et al.* Poor nutritional habits are predictors of poor outcome in very old hospitalized patients. *Am J Clin Nutr.* 2005; **82**(4): 784–91.

16. Anderson CF, Moxness K, Meister J, *et al.* The sensitivity and specificity of nutrition-related variables in relationship to duration of hospital stay and the rate of complications. *Mayo Clin Proc.* 1984; **59**(7): 477–83.

17. Cederholm T. *Topic 36: nutrition in the elderly.* ESPEN LLL Programme; 2011. Available at: http://lllnutrition.com/mod_lll/TOPIC36/m361e.htm

18. Neelemaat F, Bosmans JE, Thijs A, *et al.* Oral nutritional support in malnourished elderly decreases functional limitations with no extra costs. *Clin Nutr.* 2012; **31**(2): 183–90.

19. Beck AM, Holst M, Rasmussen HH. Oral nutritional support of older (65 years+) medical and surgical patients after discharge from hospital: systematic review and meta-analysis of randomized controlled trials. *Clin Rehabil.* 2013; **27**(1): 19–27.

20. Baldwin C, Weekes CE. Dietary advice with or without oral nutritional supplements for disease-related malnutrition in adults. *Cochrane Database Syst Rev.* 2011; (9): CD002008.

21. Lambert MA, Potter JM, McMurdo MET. Nutritional supplementation for older people. *Rev Clin Gerontol.* 2010; **20**(4): 317–26.

22. Skelly RH, Kupfer RM, Metcalfe ME, *et al.* Percutaneous endoscopic gastrostomy (PEG): change in practice since 1988. *Clin Nutr.* 2002; **21**(5): 389–94.

23. *Scoping our Practice: the 2004 report of the National Confidential Enquiry into Patient Outcome and Death.* London: NCEPOD; 2004. Available at: www.ncepod.org.uk/pdf/2004/04sum.pdf (accessed 25 March 2014).

24. Abuksis G, Mor M, Segal N, *et al.* Percutaneous endoscopic gastrostomy: high mortality rates in hospitalized patients. *Am J Gastroenterol.* 2000; **95**(1): 128–32.

25. Geeganage C, Beavan J, Ellender S, *et al.* Interventions for dysphagia and nutritional support in acute and subacute stroke. *Cochrane Database Syst Rev.* 2012; (10): CD000323.

26. Mitchell SL, Teno JM, Roy J, *et al.* Clinical and organizational factors associated with feeding tube use among nursing home residents with advanced cognitive impairment. *JAMA.* 2003; **290**(1): 73–80.

27. Royal College of Physicians and British Society of Gastroenterology. *Oral Feeding Difficulties and Dilemmas: a guide to practical care, particularly towards the end of life.* London: Royal College of Physicians; 2010.

28. Rio A, Whelan K, Goff L, *et al.* Occurrence of refeeding syndrome in adults started on artificial nutrition support: prospective cohort study. *BMJ Open.* 2013; **3**(1): e002173.

29. Fine RL. Ethical issues in artificial nutrition and hydration. *Nutr Clin Pract.* 2006; **21**(2): 118–25.

30. Klein S, Koretz RL. Nutrition support in patients with cancer: what do the data really show? *Nutr Clin Pract* 1994; **9**(3): 91–100.

31. Watson R. Measuring feeding difficulty in patients with dementia: perspectives and problems. *J Adv Nurs* 1993; **18**(1): 25–31.

32. Mitchell SL, Kiely DK, Lipsitz LA. The risk factors and impact on survival of feeding tube placement in nursing home residents with severe cognitive impairment. *Arch Intern Med.* 1997; **157**(3): 327–2.

33. www.gmc-uk.org

34. www.bma.org.uk
35. *Airedale NHS Trust v Bland* [1993] 1 All ER 821.
36. Neuberger J, Guthrie C, Aaronovitch D, *et al. More Care, Less Pathway: a review of the Liverpool Care Pathway.* London: Williams Lea; 2013.
37. McNabney MK, Beers MH, Siebens H. Surrogate decision-makers' satisfaction with the placement of feeding tubes in elderly patients. *J Am Geriatr Soc.* 1994; **42**(2): 161–8.
38. Van Rosendaal GM, Verhoef MJ, Kinsella TD. Patient and surrogate decisions re percutaneous endoscopic gastrotomy (PEG) placement. *Am J Gastroenterol.* 1997; **92**: 1665.
39. Kwok T, Twinn S, Yan E. The attitudes of Chinese family caregivers of older people with dementia towards life sustaining treatments. *J Advan Nurs.* 2007; **58**(3): 256–62.
40. O'Brien LA, Siegert EA, Grisso JA, *et al.* Tube feeding preferences among nursing home residents. *J Gen Intern Med.* 1997; **12**(6): 364–71.
41. Ouslander JG, Tymchuk AJ, Krynski MD. Decisions about enteral tube feeding among the elderly. *J Am Geriatr Soc.* 1993; **41**(1): 70–7.
42. Danis M, Southerland LI, Garrett JM, *et al.* A prospective study of advance directives for life-sustaining care. *N Engl J Med.* 1991; **324**(13): 882–8.
43. Schostak RZ. Jewish ethical guidelines for resuscitation and artificial nutrition and hydration of the dying elderly. *J Med Ethics.* 1994; **20**(2): 93–100.
44. Harris J. *The Value of Life.* London: Routledge; 1985.

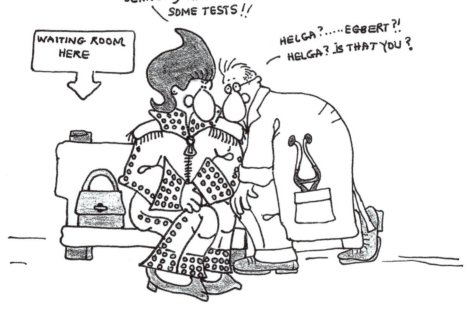

CHAPTER 5

Communication

Premila Fade, David Oliver and Philippa Gee

WHY COMMUNICATION IS IMPORTANT

Effective communication between professionals and patients is an essential building block of good medical practice. The latest edition of Good Medical Practice[1] from the General Medical Council includes a duty to 'work in partnership with patients'. Over the last 100 years the duty of care has evolved from the doctor deciding what was best to a new model of shared decision-making. Respect for patients' right to make their own decisions is now regarded as the cornerstone of beneficent care. In order to facilitate joint decision-making and promote autonomy, doctors must be able to communicate well. Doctors must listen to patients, respond to their concerns and give them information they want or need in a way that they can understand.[2]

By offering information and choices the patient is empowered to make decisions about his or her own healthcare supported by the professionals. The common law on consent to treatment,[3] the Mental Capacity Act 2005[4] and the Adults with Incapacity (Scotland) Act 2000[5] all emphasise adequate information as an essential precondition for informed decision-making. The parliamentary inquiry into the human rights of older people in healthcare[6] identified inadequate communication as a potential threat to article 3 (the right to prohibition of cruel or degrading treatment) and article 14 (the right to freedom from discrimination) under the European Convention on Human Rights 2008.[7]

GOOD COMMUNICATION

Good communication includes a duty to offer patients information on diagnosis, prognosis and treatment options, including limits of knowledge, implications and side effects of treatment, alternatives and giving patients the opportunity to ask questions. Older patients have identified these elements as key. In studies on older people's views on end-of-life care,[8] many older people wanted active involvement in planning their own treatment. The authors stress that good communication is key to achieving this. Other studies have shown that better communication may also aid concordance with medical treatment.[9,10]

Good reciprocal communication involves establishing a relationship in which patients feel empowered to ask questions or raise concerns of their own. They should be able to decide the amount of detail and style of information they want, have control over decision-making, including any delegation and involvement of family members, and in some cases may wish to be shielded from bad news. Some older people may be culturally deferential to professionals and inhibited about questioning doctors, but professionals should endeavour to find out what patients want to know and how they want it communicated.

WHAT OLDER PEOPLE WANT

Older people want to be seen as individuals, not as patient X in bed Y with condition Z. Being in a hospital bed in a hospital nightgown can make the patient feel a loss of dignity and individuality, leading to disempowerment. It is the role of the healthcare professional to engage with the individual and put him or her at the centre of the decision-making process. The patient may need time to take on board the information given, particularly if it is bad news. Not all 80-year-olds are prepared for death; many need help coming to terms with disability and life-threatening illness. The issues facing older people may be different – loss of independent living and control of their own lives are common themes, but they go through the same feelings of denial and anger as younger people and they need the same time and consideration when making life-changing decisions.

While patients' beliefs, values and culture can affect what they choose to ask and how they handle information, blanket assumptions should not be made about what individuals might want, based solely on their age, background or ethnicity. All patients should be initially encouraged to be involved in decision-making. Deliberate concealment of facts that patients want to know, or covert medication of competent people, are abuses of human rights. While these considerations matter for all patients, older people are particularly at risk of communication failure.

WHAT HAPPENS WHEN COMMUNICATION GOES WRONG?

As patients get older they are less likely to receive the right treatment, adequate information or discussion of treatment options and they may be seen as a stereotype based on a set of assumptions about age alone. If on top of this they have problems with hearing, eyesight or cognition, if they are frail and if they have no strong advocate, they are at risk of being marginalised in decisions about their treatment

When older people or their families discuss 'dignity in care',[11] many issues relate to 'insufficient choice' and 'not being listened to or treated as an individual'.[12] In European focus groups on dignity,[13] poor communication and information giving were seen by older people as key threats to their dignity. Concrete examples of dignity being compromised included being 'patronised', 'excluded from decision making' and 'treated as an object'.

The Health Service Ombudsman's report *Care and Compassion?*[14] tells the stories of 10 older people who were failed by the National Health Service (NHS): 'the investigations reveal an attitude – both personal and institutional – which fails to recognise the humanity and individuality of the people concerned and to respond to them with sensitivity, compassion and professionalism.' The majority of formal complaints about care in hospitals have a theme of poor communication. Older people often complain that they have to give the same information several times and gaps in care are often caused by poor communication between and within teams.

When communication goes wrong within institutions, when the culture of the institution is business not patients, when managers don't listen to clinical staff, the consequences are even more serious for patients. The Francis report[15] is a wake-up call to all healthcare institutions – good clinical care is the responsibility of all, from the board of directors down and must be fostered in a culture of openness within organisations that allows staff to raise issues and report clinical risks. The use of terms such as 'social admission', 'acopia' and 'bed blocker', which foster a negative attitude towards elderly patients – that they are in the wrong place or are in some way less deserving of care than other patients – also needs to change.

BARRIERS TO GOOD COMMUNICATION

Older patients are more likely to have physical disability or frailty, cognitive, hearing or visual impairment, so styles of communication and information more suited to younger, fitter patients may not always be appropriate and older patients may not be so able or ready to ask professionals for different or more information. Conversely, professionals may make patronising and ageist assumptions about the amount of information or decision-making that older people should be afforded and may fail to communicate to a degree that would seem a bare minimum in younger patients.[16] For instance, Adelman *et al.*[17] found that doctors provided more information, were more supportive and were more willing to share decision-making with younger patients than with older patients and that those patients were often reluctant to challenge them.

Professionals may also fail to see older people as individuals with individual values and communication needs, viewing them merely as a category: 'elderly people'.[8] This may be compounded by misguided attempts to 'protect' older patients from frank discussion, motivated either by paternalistic intentions to act in their 'best interests' or because the health professional fears being perceived as 'insensitive' or attracting complaints from family members.

Some staff have special difficulties in dealing with older patients from ethnic minorities – a 'disabling hesitancy'[18] – or where staff from one ethnic background are dealing with older people from another. Kai *et al.*[18] concluded that while better awareness and training might help in providing culturally sensitive communication, the onus is still on staff to treat older patients as individuals.

All these factors may result in diagnosis, treatment or future care arrangements being discussed behind the older person's back, or with the patient's family only, while the older person is effectively denied the right to determine his or her own future care or to take risks.[19,20] This can be compounded by social attitude, expectations or beliefs of the family. Families are often central to providing care for their elders, but they might believe that paternalistic, family decision-making is in the older person's best interests and that older people should not have the same right to self-determination or information about their condition as younger people.[21]

The phenomenon of 'elder speak' has been described by Williams *et al.*[22] and is something we all recognise. Staff employ infantilising language – which further reinforces dependency and helplessness – as well as insulting the older person's human dignity. As Williams *et al.*[22] concluded,

> the messages of dependence, incompetence and control to older adults by using elder-speak, a speech style similar to baby talk, that fails to communicate appropriate respect.

They describe elder speak thus:

> typically the rate of speech is slower, louder, more high pitched and using more exaggerated intonation than normal adult speech. Repetition, simple vocabulary and simple grammar are also facets of this way of talking. Diminutives and intimate terms of endearment are used rather than individuals' names.[22]

All of this reinforces the concerns raised by older people in the various reports available on dignity and rights.[5,8,12,13] Repeatedly in these reports, the issues that are raised are inadequate information, lack of time or sensitivity in the delivery of information, little consideration for the humanity of the older person and his or her individuality, inadequate mechanisms to allow older patients to express their views and preferences or to discuss their worries, and lack of respect for the decisions they wish to make over their own care.

WAYS TO IMPROVE COMMUNICATION

Much of the advice on improving communication follows from the issues already set out in this chapter. This list is not exhaustive but key points include the following.

1. *Appropriate, individualised, person-centred, non-ageist communication.* Older

people will have individual expectations, and others should not make blanket assumptions based on age, gender, illness, disability or ethnicity. Some older people freely express a wish to devolve decision-making to trusted family members or professionals or to not be burdened with much information about their treatment, illness or prognosis. In these circumstances it is misguided and maleficent to force full and frank communication. Nonetheless, the older person should retain the right to express his or her own concerns or questions or to receive 'basic' information to a degree that suits his or her individual needs. If there are cultural considerations, these should be addressed in a culturally sensitive manner. If barriers to communication are identified, then strategies should be devised in partnership with patients or carers to overcome these for that individual.

2. *Consider how, where and when communication should take place.* Ask the person who, if anyone, he or she wants to be present. Remember that curtains are not soundproof. Make sure you have enough time for the conversation and that you won't be disturbed. Think about the information you need to impart but be prepared to change and modify the information you give, depending on the patient's response (verbal and non-verbal) to you. It is normal for people to be upset by bad news but know when to stop a conversation if it is too distressing for the person. Understand the need to go back and repeat information and give the person time to ask questions, even those that may seem irrelevant.

   'Elder speak' is never acceptable, but there will be occasions where information needs to be simplified in order to make it accessible to the patient. However, the onus is on the professional to use straightforward, non-jargon-laden language to break down concepts and explain them without losing the meaning and sense – that is, to simplify but not make simplistic.

   Research has repeatedly shown that older people's preferences are generally far more in favour of full information giving than health professionals or their families anticipate (even in cultures where collectivist and family decision-making is the norm).[8,23,24] Both professionals and family can be overcautious about causing upset. Education and training can overcome such attitudes and improve skills in communication with older people in general[25] and with elders from ethnic minorities.[26]

3. *The use of written information.* This is not a substitute for adequate verbal communication, but it may help for those whose first language is not English, those with poor short-term memory or poor retention due to anxiety, and those with hearing impairment. The use of such information may increase satisfaction with care and understanding of treatment, reduce complaints, improve self-care and management and make the older patient feel more empowered, so reducing his or her anxiety or distress.[27] All patients have the right to receive a copy of clinical correspondence about them. Well-worded discharge summaries and clinic letters provide an excellent way of improving communication with the patient and his or her carers if required. Sharing information with patients suffering from chronic diseases

helps them feel part of the decision-making process and empowers them to become a partner in their own healthcare.

4. *Interpreters.* While most hospitals and primary care organisations have access to interpretation services, staff sometimes rely on family members or friends.[12] This can cause problems when there are no immediate family or friends and might potentially compromise the privacy and dignity of the older person if sensitive personal information is being shared with others merely because of the ease of an 'on hand' translator. It may be hard for those personally involved to translate impartially if they themselves have views, agendas, vested interests or control over that older person. Booking an external interpreter may sometimes be impractical where instant communication is required, but this option should always be available to older patients. If hospital staff are used as *ad hoc* interpreters, it is preferable that they are clinically trained rather than ancillary staff.

5. *Services for the hard of hearing.* The Royal National Institute for Deaf People[28] estimates that there are 123 000 deafened people aged over 16 within the UK, with the incidence of deafness increasing with age. We often fail to consider whether an older person in health or social care settings has a hearing loss, whether diagnosed or undiagnosed – with the assumption being made that the person doesn't understand, is confused or is simply being obstructive. However, the Mental Capacity Act 2005[4] states that capacity should always be assumed unless proven otherwise. Professionals have a duty to facilitate adequate understanding and information giving. This entails an obligation to perform adequate assessment and remediation if possible of any hearing loss. Deaf people who communicate using sign language can also exhibit the characteristics of aphasia following a stroke.[29] Difficulty in communicating is further compounded by the use of elder speak, as shouting can distort the pattern of speech and the use of a high-pitched tone exacerbates the situation, as the hearing loss pattern associated with ageing is so often one of high-frequency loss.[30]

6. *Patients with dysphasia.* Dysphasia or aphasia may be defined as 'a complex disorder which can affect comprehension, speech, reading and writing to varying degrees' and affects approximately one-third of stroke survivors.[31] It often coexists with other disorders such as hearing loss, visual impairment, dysarthria and dyspraxia. It is often assumed that older people with aphasia cannot understand or communicate sufficiently well to make decisions – thus increasing their exclusion and disempowerment.[32] The Connect Report[31] stated that: 'People with aphasia are frequently treated as stupid. They can feel excluded, ignored and unable to participate fully in life. And that's on top of the personal struggle of learning to live with a long term disability.'

    Older people with a possible diagnosis of aphasia should be formally assessed to determine the degree of disability and be given the chance fully to participate in any decision-making even if this requires facilitation.[33,34]

7. *Family, carers and patient advocates.* Health professionals may be suspicious

of recorded or witnessed consultations, seeing them as a breach of trust or a potential threat of litigation. However, if viewed from the patient's perspective the desire for a witness is much more understandable. The patient may be feeling scared and vulnerable; the patient may be worried that he or she won't remember to give the right information or won't remember what is said. Having a family member, carer or friend with the patient can be hugely reassuring and helpful to the healthcare professional, ensuring that information and advice are remembered accurately. Although it may alter the nature of the conversation, having a relative or patient advocate present also helps patients if they have hearing or communication problems or if English is not their first language. As long as patients agree, it is good practice to involve people close to them, bearing in mind the duty of confidentiality. This also helps carers meet the individual's care needs. Competent patients must always be offered a choice about who is involved in the discussion, and even if the patient is not competent to make healthcare decisions he or she should be asked whom he or she wants to be involved in decisions about his or her care. Recording the conversation has some advantages but may make communication more difficult. The professional is likely to be more cautious and less willing to speculate about future options or explore areas of uncertainty with the patient.

Patient advocacy services are provided by some charitable organisations and public services providers such as local authorities and NHS hospitals, in order to help individuals understand the choices available to them and to represent their views and concerns. Legally, patient advocates (even independent mental capacity advocates appointed under the Mental Capacity Act 2005[4]) have no formal decision-making powers, but they can help the decision-making process by facilitating communication. Advocates should be properly trained and, whether or not an advocate is present, health professionals should, where possible, still communicate directly with the patient, as patients accompanied by advocates or carers feel excluded if health professionals fail to speak directly to them. There are times when an independent advocate with no emotional investment in the situation is the most appropriate person to support a person making difficult decisions. However, roles must be clearly defined and everyone involved needs to be aware of the scope and limits of advocates' powers.

DEMENTIA AND COGNITIVE IMPAIRMENT

Once patients have been given a diagnosis of dementia, assumptions may be made about their ability to process information and only limited attempts may be made to communicate fully and explain treatment decisions properly. Healthcare professionals may misguidedly communicate instead with relatives and carers, leaving the patient excluded from important decisions about his or her future care. Patient groups[35,36] have expressed concerns that staff automatically make assumptions and set low expectations about the ability of older patients with dementia to communicate or make care decisions, even though the literature on mental capacity[37,38] and the legal tests[4] make it clear that the mere presence of the diagnosis does not make the older person incapable of decision-making or of some involvement in planning his or her own care. It is not uncommon for professionals to question decision-making capacity just because an older person makes a decision they consider unwise. However, it is also common for family members and carers to feel excluded from medical consultations and decision-making, which makes their role as carer more difficult. Medical professionals may be so concerned with confidentiality that they fail to even talk to relatives, which may mean that important information is missed. It is important to remember that seeking more information from others does not necessarily breach the confidentiality of the individual. The duty of confidentiality is of course important, but where capacity is borderline and when the person requires support from his or her family to function, it is much more helpful to encourage the patient to include the family in healthcare discussions and decisions. A different philosophical view about the importance of confidentiality is articulated in the Nuffield report on dementia, which sees people with dementia as embedded in their social world and argues that respecting their autonomy necessitates involvement and recognition of the interests of family and carers.

The Mental Capacity Act 2005 was designed to protect vulnerable adults from paternalistic decision-making. The presumption of capacity cannot be refuted merely on the basis of a diagnosis of mental impairment or mental illness, an unwise decision or refusal of treatment. The Mental Capacity Act 2005 also makes it clear that capacity is decision specific and must be assessed using the two-stage test. Stage 1 asks if the person is suffering from a disorder or impairment of the mind or brain. Only if stage 1 is positive can the professional move on to stage 2, which assesses comprehension of information (and retention for as long as it takes to come to a decision), decision-making and communication. Even when assessment of capacity shows the person does not have capacity, the best interests checklist is there to ensure the person's current views, previously expressed views, values and beliefs are all taken into account. Relatives, carers or others close to the person must also be consulted to throw light on what the incapacitated person would have wanted. The final point on the checklist is often forgotten but is extremely important, particularly in light of the Bournewood ruling from the European Court of Human Rights[39] and subsequent Deprivation of Liberty Safeguards amendment to the Mental Capacity Act 2005 in the Mental Health Act 2007, which is that the least restrictive option should be chosen. The European Court of Human Rights ruled that adults with mental incapacity should not be treated in a way that deprives them of access to their family and social network unless absolutely necessary; they should have a mechanism of appeal (or mechanism for appeal on their behalf) if they are deprived of their liberty (this led to the Deprivation of Liberty Safeguards amendment to the Mental Capacity Act 2005); and they should be allowed as much autonomy over their own care as is feasible.[40]

If it is decided that the person does lack capacity for the issue at hand, then final responsibility for making the treatment decision rests with the health professional in charge, who must act in the patient's best interests. When invoking 'best interests', the Department of Health[20] and the best practice guidance accompanying the Mental Capacity Act 2005[4] prioritise communication, encouraging the following elements:

➤ doing whatever is practical to help the person participate in decision-making
➤ identifying factors that the person would take into account if acting for him- or herself
➤ reflecting his or her known wishes and any statement made before capacity was lost
➤ identifying the values that would be likely to influence the decision if the patient had capacity
➤ avoiding assumptions about his or her best interests based on age, appearance, condition or behaviour
➤ considering whether he or she is likely to regain capacity
➤ consulting other people where possible for their views.

Relatives often find the best interests decision-making process confusing; they may mistakenly believe that they have the right or responsibility to decide what treatment is given or withheld, and this can add to their anxiety and distress. The healthcare professional needs to communicate sensitively with the relatives (who may themselves be elderly and vulnerable) and explain how treatment decisions are made.

CONFIDENTIALITY AND INFORMATION SHARING

We have discussed in this chapter the need for adequate, appropriate and individualised communication with older people. However, in many cases where their needs are complex it is impossible to plan their care without sharing information and discussing details of their case. Often, it will be in an older person's interests to discuss aspects of his or her care with family or friends, and this should be encouraged unless the individual objects. Where optimum care of an older person requires input from a range of agencies and professionals, a degree of information sharing between professionals and agencies is desirable and inevitable.

Reports have shown that many older people actively wish information to be shared between agencies and resent having to repeat the same information to several professionals.[39,41–43] They are usually happy to have information shared, so long as it is between individuals acting for their welfare. For all this, there are caveats and concerns around information sharing.

Areas of the law relevant to information sharing in the care of older people

➤ *Data Protection Act 1998.*[44] This requires organisations fairly and lawfully to process information on patients and provides that patients must be informed about what information about them is being processed. The processing must meet legal standards for confidentiality. The Act also requires organisations sharing information to share the *minimum amount necessary* and to retain it only for as long as is needed.

➤ All *identifiable, patient-related* information is subject to a professional duty of confidentiality. Electronically stored or written information must be protected and stored securely. Any confidential conversations should be conducted out of earshot of others. However, there are exceptions to these rules:
— where the patient gives consent to others being informed
— where the law requires disclosure of information
— where there is an overriding public interest.

➤ *Human Rights Act 1998, article 8.*[45] This articulates a right to 'respect for private and family life', though this right is not absolute and may be derogated from where necessary in a democratic society in the interests of national security, public safety, economic well-being or the prevention of crime.

➤ *Common law.* This reinforces the view for various judgments that information may be disclosed with patient consent, where there is a public interest or where the law requires it.[3]

➤ *NHS care record guarantee.* This sets out rules governing information held electronically by NHS care records, including patients' access to their own records and control over access by others.

➤ *Professional codes of conduct.* These set out duties around confidentiality, privacy and data sharing.[46,47]

➤ *Internal policies of employing organisations.* All patients who are mentally competent have a right to object to the disclosure of information that they provide in confidence.

Patient consent to disclosure between professionals is usually implicit; that is, it is assumed that patients understand that information about them is shared in order to provide healthcare. This is a reasonable assumption because patients see doctors and nurses discussing their care and notes being written and shared. However, patients may not realise that information is shared with other agencies and they should be told if this is necessary. When health professionals make implicit assumptions, they must demonstrate that they were acting reasonably and in good faith in assuming consent.

INFORMATION SHARING WITH PATIENTS' RELATIVES

This is a common area of misunderstanding and conflict between healthcare staff and patients' relatives. Relatives and carers often object to being excluded from day-to-day discussion of a patient's care. In complaints from the relatives of older patients, concerns are often raised that 'we were given no information/ were not told what was going on'. Many older patients *do* want their families to be kept informed and patients often assume that their spouse or other close relatives will automatically be included in information sharing, but all patients are entitled to confidentiality and should first be asked about how they want information shared with other people, and with whom.

Doctors do not have a right to inform relatives when the patient is lucid and is fully able to discuss his or her own care; they are governed by a strong duty of confidentiality. However, this same patient although compos mentis may be anxious and worried, which will affect the patient's ability to take in the information given to him or her, which in turn may hamper his or her compliance with treatment, and the patient may be dependent on family members for day-to-day support or care. In this scenario the autonomy of the patient is best promoted by encouraging him or her to share information and medical decision-making. Nevertheless, professionals should not assume that patients are necessarily on good terms with their relatives or want their relatives to have confidential information. The best course of action is to ask patients with whom and when they would like information to be shared.

A further complicated problem arises when relatives insist that *they alone* be given information without its being shared with the patient – this may happen when bad news is expected and the relatives make this plea on the basis that the patient would be too distressed by the bad news or that the patient would not want to know. However, this should be resisted – as stated earlier, generally patients want more information even when the news is bad. Uncertainty is generally more frightening than knowing, and knowledge is essential in order to plan for the future. In this situation it is best to get everyone to communicate with one another together. The relatives may well have the patient's best interests at heart but may in fact be mistaking their own grief and distress for that of their relative.

The law and information sharing with patients' relatives and friends

Information on mentally competent patients should not be shared with family members without the patient's consent. It is *for the patient to decide* what information is shared and with whom. Where patients lack capacity, it is usual to assume that they would want those close to them to be informed, unless there is clear evidence that they would not want information shared or it becomes evident that to share information would put the patient at risk.

INFORMATION SHARING WITH OTHER PROFESSIONALS

Poor communication between care providers is a frequent cause of serious adverse events in healthcare. A breakdown in the communication of data, such as investigation results, can be due to a lack of clarity or prior agreement about who has ownership of the data and the responsibility for ensuring that other health professionals are kept informed. Help the Aged[8] gathered examples of lack of coordination and communication between healthcare staff or between healthcare providers and social care staff – especially when older patients were discharged from hospital or transferred from one type of care to another. Evidence of poor communication between health staff also occurred in hospital settings when the health professionals providing specialised care had been informed about the patient's need for that specialised treatment but had not been given other relevant information, such as the fact that the patient was blind or suffered from dementia. The National Institute for Health and Care Excellence has particularly highlighted the need for well-organised dementia care.[48] Research also shows that 'much of the distress experienced by people with dementia and their families can be prevented by primary care working closely with nurse practitioners, social services, and community and voluntary services'.[49]

Partnership working across primary care, secondary care, community services and with social care is essential for older people and requires excellent communication and information sharing between sectors that often have their own IT systems and patient records that don't interface or communicate automatically. Information needs to be shared in such a way that all parties can understand and contribute, and here again it is important not to miss out family carers, who often complain that they get less information than professional carers but that they do the same job.

The law and information sharing with other professionals

In the absence of evidence to the contrary, patients are generally assumed to have consented to information being shared with other professionals for the purpose of the care they receive, so long as that information is both *necessary* and *relevant*. It is important that patients know what information will be shared and with whom. This has implications for older people with *multi-agency working*, including social services, housing associations, voluntary agencies, and so forth. Health professionals should discuss with patients from the outset the desirability of such information sharing.

Other relevant specific points of law around data sharing
The law and secondary use of information

If information is being used for research, audit or service planning, it may be disclosed to an appropriate authority if:
➤ it is sufficiently anonymised
➤ it is required by law
➤ it is with explicit consent
➤ health professionals are satisfied that the patient is aware of its use and has not objected (implied consent)
➤ health professionals are satisfied that legal and professional criteria for disclosure 'in public interest' have been met.

The law and data sharing in official complaints

Here it is implicit that a complaint cannot be satisfactorily answered without adequate access to information, although there is guidance from health departments on confidentiality in complaints.

Summary of the legal position on information sharing

➤ Patients must be properly informed about the use of information.
➤ Consent should be sought for disclosure of personal information.
➤ Occasionally where consent cannot be obtained, information may be disclosed where the law requires it or where there is a public interest.
➤ Health professionals should anonymise information wherever possible.
➤ Health professionals should disclose the minimum amount of information needed to achieve the purpose.
➤ When competent patients refuse disclosure, their wishes should be respected.
➤ Health professionals should always be able to justify the reason for their disclosure.

CONCLUSION

Good communication between clinicians, patients, their families, carers and other professionals or agencies is crucial in the delivery of high-quality care. This is all the more important when the older patients are frail, disabled, have sensory or cognitive impairment or complex needs. Yet it is often with these very patients that communication and confidentiality can be compromised. High-quality care should provide individually tailored communication that respects human dignity, as well as known attitudes and beliefs, and which gives the patient autonomous control over decisions affecting his or her healthcare. While the role of family and carers is often crucial to safe care of such older patients, it is very important that the wishes and views of older people are not bypassed in favour of family members or carers. It is also true that effective care often requires communication between agencies and professionals. Nonetheless, in sharing such information, it is important that the older person retains some control over the extent and detail of such sharing and that information is shared only to the extent that it will benefit the care of the older person in question. An awareness of these issues and the ethical and legal considerations that surround them is crucial in the day-to-day clinical and social care of older people.

Doctors have a duty of care that encompasses more than the patient in front of us; we have a responsibility to promote the wider interests of our patients, to ensure that elderly patients receive the same standards of care and compassion as younger patients. We have an ethical duty to speak up for their rights and needs within the organisations in which we work and the wider healthcare community.[50]

REFERENCES

1. General Medical Council. *Good Medical Practice.* Manchester: GMC; 2013.
2. Gillon R. Medical ethics: four principles plus attention to scope. *BMJ.* 1994; **309**(6948): 184–8.
3. Mason JK, McCall Smith RA, Laurie GT. Consent to treatment. In: Mason JK, McCall Smith RA, Laurie GT, editors. *Law and Medical Ethics.* 6th ed. London: LexisNexis; 2002. pp. 309–64.
4. *Mental Capacity Act 2005.* London: Office of Public Sector Information. Available at: www.opsi.gov.uk/ACTS/acts2005/ukpga_20050009_en_1 (accessed 14 April 2009).
5. *Adults with Incapacity (Scotland) Act 2000.* London: Office of Public Sector Information. Available at: www.opsi.gov.uk/legislation/scotland/acts2000/asp_20000004_en_1 (accessed 14 April 2009).
6. House of Lords, House of Commons Joint Committee on Human Rights. *The Human Rights of Older People in Healthcare.* London: Office of Public Sector Information; 2007.
7. *Human Rights Act 1998.* London: Office of Public Sector Information. Available at: www.opsi.gov.uk/ACTS/acts1998/ukpga_19980042_en_1 (accessed 14 April 2009).
8. Help the Aged. *Listening to Older People: opening the door for older people to explore end of life issues.* London: Help the Aged; 2006.
9. British Medical Association. *Evidence Based Prescribing.* London: BMJ Publishing; 2007.
10. Engova D, Duggan C, MacCallum P, *et al.* Patients' understanding and perceptions of treatment as determinants of adherence to warfarin treatment. *Int J Pharm Pract.* 2002; **10**(Suppl. 1): R69.
11. Aitken M. The dignity and privacy of patients. *J Royal Soc Med.* 2008; **101**(3): 108–9.
12. Healthcare Commission. *Caring for Dignity: a national report on dignity in care for older people while in hospital.* London: Healthcare Commission; 2007.
13. Woolhead G, Calnan M, Dieppe P, *et al.* Dignity in older age: what do older people in the United Kingdom think? *Age Ageing.* 2004; **33**(2): 165–70.
14. Parliamentary and Health Service Ombudsman. *Care and Compassion? Report of the Health Service Ombudsman on ten investigations into NHS care of older people.* London: TSO; 2011.
15. Francis R. *Independent Inquiry into Care Provided by Mid Staffordshire NHS Foundation Trust January 2005–March 2009.* Vol. 375. London: TSO; 2010.
16. Oliver D. Acopia and social admissions are not diagnoses: why older people deserve better. *J Royal Soc Med.* 2008; **101**(4): 168–74.
17. Adelman R, Greene M, Charon R, *et al.* Content of elderly patient–physician interviews in the medical primary care encounter. *Commun Res.* 1992; **19**(3): 370–80.
18. Kai J, Beavan J, Faull C, *et al.* Professional uncertainty and disempowerment responding to ethnic diversity in healthcare: a qualitative study. *PLoS Med.* 2007; **4**(11): e323.
19. Counsel and Care. *The Right to Take Risks.* London: Counsel and Care; 1993.
20. Department of Health. *Independence, Choice and Risk: a guide to best practice in supported decision making.* London: DH; 2007.
21. Edwards H, Chapman H. Communicating in family aged care dyads: the influence of role expectation. *Qual Ageing.* 2004; **5**(2): 3–9.
22. Williams K, Kemper S, Hummert ML. Enhancing communication with older adults: overcoming elderspeak. *J Gerontol Nurs.* 2004; **30**(10): 17–25.

23. Ajaj A, Singh MP, Abdulla AJJ. Should elderly patients be told they have cancer? Questionnaire survey of older people. *BMJ*. 2001; **323**: 1160.

24. Scriven MW. Patients' attitudes towards 'do not attempt resuscitation' status. *J Med Ethics*. 2008; **34**: 624–6.

25. Baltes MM, Neumann EM, Zank S. Maintenance and rehabilitation of independence in old age: an intervention programme for staff. *Psychol Aging*. 1994; **9**(2): 179–88.

26. Cancer Research UK. *Professionals Responding to Cancer and Ethnic Diversity (PROCEED)*. London: Cancer Research UK; 2006.

27. Payne SA. Balancing information needs: dilemmas in producing patient information leaflets. *Health Informatics J*. 2002; **8**(4): 174–9.

28. Royal National Institute for Deaf People. *Impact Report*. London: RNID; 2008. Videos available at: www.youtube.com/playlist?list=PL3821E93E24267C59 (accessed 23 March 2014).

29. Royal College of Speech and Language Therapists. *Communicating Quality 3*. London: RCSLT; 2006. Available at: www.rcslt.org/speech_and_language_therapy/standards/CQ3_pdf (accessed 23 March 2014).

30. Kulkarni K, Hartley DE. Recent advances in hearing restoration. *J Royal Soc Med*. 2008; **101**(3): 116–24.

31. Connect. *No Longer Invisible: Connect's impact report*. London: Connect; 2006/07. Available at: www.ukconne ct.org/upload/Connect%20IR%200607%20FINAL%20VERSION.pdf (accessed 23 March 2014).

32. Hilari K. Predictors of health-related quality of life in people with chronic aphasia. *Aphasiology*. 2000; **17**(14): 365–81.

33. Royal College of Physicians of London, Intercollegiate Working Party on Stroke. *National Clinical Guidelines for Stroke*. London: Royal College of Physicians; 2008.

34. Rose M. The effectiveness of aphasia-friendly principles for printed health education materials for people with aphasia following stroke. *Aphasiology*. 2003; **17**(10): 947–63.

35. The Scottish Dementia Working Group is an independent group run by people with dementia. Available at: www.alzscot.org/campaigning/scottish_dementia_working_group (accessed 23 March 2014).

36. Department of Health. *The National Dementia Strategy*. London: Department of Health; 2008. Available at: www.gov.uk/government/uploads/system/uploads/attachment_data/file/168220/dh_094051.pdf (accessed 23 March 2014).

37. Alderson P, Goodey C. Theories of consent. *BMJ*. 1998; **317**(7168): 1313–15.

38. Grisso T, Appelbaum P. Comparisons of standards for assessing patients' capacities to make a treatment decision. *Am J Psychiatry*. 1995; **152**(7): 1033–7.

39. Department of Health. *Briefing Sheet. Mental Health Bill. Bournewood safeguards*. London: DH; 2006.

40. Harwood RH, Stewart R, Bartlett B. Safeguarding the rights of patients who lack capacity in general hospitals: do the Bournewood proposals for England and Wales help or hinder? *Age Ageing*. 2007; **36**: 120–1.

41. Department of Health. *National Service Framework for Older People*. London: DH; 2001. Available at: www.dh.gov.uk/en/Publicationsandstatistics/Publications/PublicationsPolicyAndGuidance/DH_4003066 (accessed 14 April 2009).

42. Healthcare Commission, Audit Commission, Commission for Social Care and Inspection. *Living Well in Late Life*. London: Office of Public Sector Information; 2006.

43. *With Respect to Old Age: the Royal Commission into Long Term Care for Older People.* London: HMSO; 1999.

44. *Data Protection Act 1998.* London: Office of Public Sector Information. Available at: www.legislation.gov.uk/ukpga/1998/29/contents (accessed 23 March 2014).

45. *Human Rights Act 1998.* London: Office of Public Sector Information. Available at: www.opsi.gov.uk/ACTS/acts1998/ukpga_19980042_en_1 (accessed 14 April 2009).

46. General Medical Council. The duties of a doctor registered with the General Medical Council. In: General Medical Council. *Good Medical Practice.* Manchester: GMC; 2013.

47. Nursing and Midwifery Council. *The Code: standards for conduct, performance and ethics for nurses and midwives.* London: NMC; 2010. Available at www.nmc-uk.org/Documents/Standards/nmcTheCodeStandardsofConductPerformanceAndEthicsForNursesAndMidwives_TextVersion.pdf (accessed 23 March 2014).

48. National Institute for Health and Clinical Excellence. *Dementia: supporting people with dementia and their carers in health and social care.* NICE clinical guideline 42. London: NICE; 2006. Available at: www.nice.org.uk/guidance/cg42 (accessed 14 April 2009).

49. Downs M, Bowers B. Caring for people with dementia. *BMJ.* 2008; **336**(7638): 225–6.

50. Royal College of Physicians. *Putting Patients First: realising Francis's vision.* London: RCP; 2013.

CHAPTER 6

Cardiopulmonary resuscitation

Gurcharan S Rai

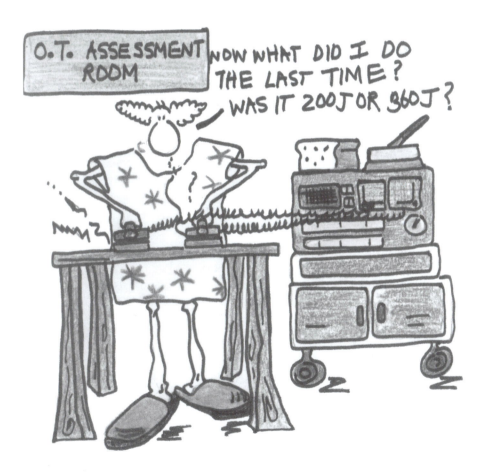

INTRODUCTION

Cardiopulmonary resuscitation (CPR) is routinely attempted when hospital inpatients suffer cardiac arrest, unless a specific decision is made in advance to withhold it. However, such 'do not attempt resuscitation' (DNAR) or 'do not attempt cardiopulmonary resuscitation' decisions can be controversial. In the UK, there has been considerable media and public concern about DNAR decisions following several high-profile cases, and there have been demands for more openness and transparency in the decision-making process. In 2007, the British Medical Association, the Royal College of Nursing and the Resuscitation Council (UK) updated their guidelines on DNAR decision-making to take into consideration the Mental Capacity Act 2005 (England and Wales), the Adult with Incapacity (Scotland) Act 2000 and provisions of the Human Rights Act 1998. The articles of the Human Rights Act 1998 that pertain to decision-making about resuscitation include:

➤ article 2 – the right to protection for life
➤ article 3 – the right to freedom from inhuman or degrading treatment
➤ article 8 – the right to respect for privacy and family life
➤ article 10 – the right to hold opinions and receive information
➤ article 14 – the right to be free from discriminatory practices (e.g. ageism).

The guidelines recognise the following points.
1. The goal of medicine is not just to prolong life at all costs.
2. It is lawful to withhold CPR on the basis that to do so would be in the patient's best interests, where consideration has been given to relevant medical factors and the quality of life of patients who lack capacity.
3. A competent patient has the right to accept or refuse resuscitation after he or she has been fully informed of its benefits and risks.
4. It is not necessary to initiate discussion with patients if there is no reason to believe that they are likely to suffer a cardiopulmonary arrest or they do not wish to have CPR or they will not survive cardiopulmonary arrest even if CPR is attempted.
5. Doctors should always be prepared to discuss DNAR decisions with competent patients and they should usually consult other staff.
6. Under the Human Rights Act 1998, relatives and carers have the right to information with the consent of the competent patient. Their role is to help the doctor in decision-making and to reflect what the incompetent patient would choose in the current circumstances, if the patient were competent. They do not have the right to demand or reject resuscitation or a DNAR order.
7. In the case of adults who lack capacity, the clinician should use the guidance included in the Mental Capacity Act 2005 in assessing best interests.
8. The overall responsibility for decisions about CPR and DNAR rests with the consultant or general practitioner in charge of the patient's care.
9. Decisions about CPR must be reviewed regularly, especially when the patient's condition changes.

MAKING A DNAR DECISION

When should a DNAR decision be made and for which patients?

Predicting which hospital inpatients might require DNAR decisions is a difficult task. Most of those patients who survive CPR attempts have a cardiac arrest within the first couple of days of hospital admission, but at this time many patients may be too ill to be involved in decision-making. Studies suggest that around 40% of acute medical inpatients may lack capacity to make such decisions. A recent National Confidential Enquiry into Patient Outcome and Death report (Time to Intervene) recommended that an explicit decision about CPR be made in all acutely ill patients as early as possible during their hospital stay. The Resuscitation Council (UK) in association with the British Medical Association and the Royal College of Nursing are reviewing their joint statement and 'quality standards for cardiopulmonary resuscitation practice and training'.

At the present time it is considered appropriate to make a DNAR decision in the following five circumstances:
1. where the clinical outcome, including the likelihood of successfully starting the patient's heart and breathing, is poor
2. where CPR is not in accord with the recorded, sustained wishes of a competent patient
3. where successful CPR is likely to be followed by a length and quality of life that would be unacceptable to the patient
4. where the patient already has a poor quality of life and does not wish to have his or her life prolonged
5. where the patient has made an advance decision refusing CPR under a clearly defined situation and wishes; however, if no advance explicit decision has been made about CPR and the wishes of the patient are unknown and cannot be ascertained, doctors should make reasonable effort to attempt to resuscitate the patient.

Who should make the decision?

'Senior experienced doctors' should take responsibility for decision-making. In hospital practice in the UK, this is likely to mean those at consultant or specialist registrar level, or those with similar experience. In some circumstances it may be necessary for more junior staff to make decisions, such as when they are the most senior doctor attending a deteriorating patient who has a very clear advance refusal of life-sustaining treatment. In such circumstances, good practice guidance suggests that more senior doctors are informed of the decision as soon as practicably possible.

If there is doubt or disagreement about decisions, full active treatment should be given until the situation is resolved.

DISCUSSION WITH THE PATIENT AND FAMILIES

Competent patients

All DNAR orders for competent patients should be discussed with the patients, unless they indicate that they do not want this. It may be acceptable to avoid such discussion if it is considered that this is likely to be harmful to the patient (i.e. cause anxiety and distress). Doctors who avoid discussing decisions with competent patients in these circumstances must be able to explain their decisions on the basis that the potential for harm justifies excluding the patient from the process. If the patient indicates that he or she does not wish to discuss this, his or her decision should be respected.

Discussion of CPR should focus on:

➤ the risks and benefits of CPR for the individual, with a realistic estimate of the chances of starting the heart and breathing for a sustained period and the likelihood of long-term survival and associated morbidity

➤ the patient's wishes, feelings, beliefs and values

➤ the patient's human rights, including the right to life and the right to be free from degrading treatment

➤ the likelihood of the patient experiencing severe unmanageable pain, suffering or other adverse effects.

If a patient becomes incompetent after he or she has made a decision, then the patient's original decision stands, provided that the circumstances that have arisen are as envisaged by the patient when he or she made the decision. Clearly if a long period of time has passed since the initial decision, then there is a risk that circumstances may have changed significantly. It is recommended that DNAR orders and other such decisions are reviewed regularly to avoid this problem.

Incompetent patients

Before discussing this it is important to remember that a doctor must work on the presumption that every adult patient has the capacity to make decisions about his or her care and treatment. The doctor must not assume that a patient lacks capacity to make a decision solely because of his or her age, disability, appearance, behaviour, medical condition (including mental illness), beliefs, apparent inability to communicate or because he or she makes a decision that others disagree with or consider unwise. Doctor must also consider the following points.

➤ Whether it is likely that the person will at some time have capacity in relation to CPR decision; and if it appears likely that the person will, when that is likely to be.

➤ The doctor must, so far as is reasonably practicable, permit and encourage the person to participate, or to improve his or her ability to participate, as fully as possible in the decision-making.

➤ In considering whether DNAR is in the best interests of the person concerned, the doctor must not be motivated by a desire to bring about the person's death.

If the patient lacks capacity and has not left clear instruction, in the form of an advance decision or nomination of a proxy decision-maker using the lasting power of attorney, or does not have a court-appointed deputy or guardian, then the doctor has an obligation to act 'in the best interests' of the patient (*see* Table 6.1). In practice, this means discussing the decision (where practicable) with other professionals involved in the patient's care, the patient's family, others close to the patient and any formal or informal carers.

TABLE 6.1 Factors to be taken into account when making a 'best interests' assessment

- Identifying things that an individual would take into account if acting for him- or herself
- The patient's past and present expressed wishes
- The patient's beliefs and values
- Views of family, friends, carers and general practitioner regarding what the patient would have wanted for him- or herself
- Views of an independent mental capacity advocate if the patient has no family or friends

Such discussions should not focus on asking family and friends to act as proxy decision-makers (the doctor still has an obligation to make the decision) but rather should seek to determine the patient's best interests. To do this, the doctor might ask about the patient's previously held views and beliefs or about any statements that the patient may have made in the past. Questions such as 'What do you think your father would have wanted for himself if he knew he was going to be in these circumstances?' may be useful in the discussion. If there is no family, friend or carer to consult, then doctors must appoint an independent mental capacity advocate to assist with his or her decision-making.

DIFFERENCES OF OPINION BETWEEN PATIENTS AND THEIR FAMILIES

Conflict between the view of patients and that of their families can arise under several circumstances.

1. If a competent patient refuses to give permission to doctors to discuss his or her medical condition and treatment options – under these circumstances, the patient's views prevail.
2. If the decision made by the competent patient is different to that suggested by the relatives – under these circumstances, the physician should facilitate a discussion between them with the aim of reaching a common understanding of the rights of competent patients to exercise their autonomy.
3. Families sometimes question patients' competence (or doctors' assessment of this), especially perhaps when they disagree with DNAR decisions that apparently competent patients have made. In these circumstances doctors

should carefully record their assessment of competence using a standardised approach and the questions suggested by the guidance to the Mental
Capacity Act 2005. Second clinical opinions can help to clarify the situation in disputes around competence.
4. If there is no resolution after all the aforementioned avenues have been
explored then it is appropriate to seek a legal opinion.

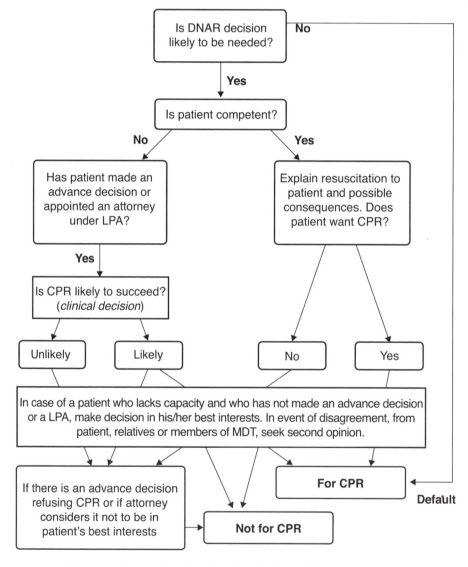

FIGURE 6.1 Suggested resuscitation algorithm for hospital admission
(CPR = cardiopulmonary resuscitation; DNAR = 'do not attempt resuscitation';
LPA = lasting power of attorney; MDT = multidisciplinary team)

WHEN THE SUCCESS OF CPR IS CONSIDERED TO BE POOR

Although the term 'medical futility' is not included in the 2007 guideline, it is recognised that a clinical team need not attempt CPR if the team believes that it will not restart the heart and maintain breathing or if a patient is in his or her final stages of a terminal illness. If, however, a person wishes to delay death, even for a short period, this wish should be respected provided this has been made after full, accurate information has been given to the patient about the length of survival that realistically can be expected.

CASE 6.1

Mrs A, aged 84 years, was admitted to hospital with intracerebral bleeding following a fall. She had a past history of manic-depressive illness and required supervision from her husband for basic activities of daily living. At the time of admission she had a Glasgow Coma Scale score of 9/15, and she had spontaneous movement in the left arm and left leg but no movements in the right leg and right arm and bilateral plantar extensor responses. The duty medical registrar who assessed Mrs A made a DNAR decision on the grounds that CPR was unlikely to be successful and would not be in Mrs A's best interests. However, when he discussed this with Mrs A's husband and daughter, they demanded that she should be resuscitated. Despite a prolonged discussion, no consensus could be reached.

A second clinical opinion was sought from an experienced colleague. He agreed that CPR was unlikely to be successful and undertook further discussion with the family. He discovered that they feared that a DNAR order would mean Mrs A's being denied access to tube feeding, antibiotics and other life-prolonging treatment. When it was explained to them that this was not the case, they accepted the need for a DNAR order.

Comments
- Patients' families and some professionals, may believe that a DNAR decision automatically precludes other life-prolonging treatments. DNAR decisions refer to CPR only.
- Second clinical opinions can help to clarify situations and resolve differences of opinion with families.
- It is often difficult to be sure that CPR will not succeed unless patients are clearly in the last few hours of life. If there is a degree of uncertainty about this, and there is no other basis for making a DNAR decision, then the patient should remain for CPR until the situation becomes clearer.

CASE 6.2

An 84-year-old woman with long-standing rheumatoid arthritis and who required a considerable amount of aid and support from the community services was admitted with a 1-week history of nausea and vomiting. She was somewhat dehydrated but otherwise clinically stable. She seemed mildly confused and her Abbreviated Mental Test score was 7/10. No family were present when she was admitted. The middle-grade doctor who admitted her concluded that it would be difficult to resuscitate her successfully should she have a cardiorespiratory arrest and so recorded DNAR in her notes. He did not discuss this with the patient.

Comments

Several issues arise from this case.

- It appears that an assumption was made that the patient was incompetent. While many acute medical inpatients may be incompetent, a competence assessment should be documented if decisions about life-prolonging treatment are being made.
- If decisions are being made about patients who are assumed to be incompetent, then efforts should be made to elicit the opinions of family and friends around their best interests.
- Doctors in training or those who are relatively inexperienced should be cautious about making decisions about CPR, or other life-prolonging treatments, without reference to senior colleagues.
- Unless the clinical situation is grave, or rapidly deteriorating, then it is often best to avoid making DNAR decisions early after admission when the information available is likely to be incomplete.

FURTHER READING

- Appelbaum PS. Clinical practice. Assessment of patients' competence to consent to treatment. *N Engl J Med.* 2007; **357**(18): 1834–80.
- British Medical Association. *The Impact of the Human Rights Act 1998 on Medical Decision Making.* London: BMA; 2000.
- British Medical Association. *Decisions Relating to Cardiopulmonary Resuscitation: a joint statement from the British Medical Association, the Resuscitation Council (UK) and the Royal College of Nursing.* London: BMA; 2007.
- *Care Quality Commission: supporting note on do not attempt resuscitation (DNAR) for assessors and inspectors.* Available at: www.cqc.org.uk/sites/default/files/media/documents/20111028_100483_v2.00_supporting_note_on_resuscitation_-_staffing_support_for_publication (accessed 25 March 2014).
- Ethics Department. *Decision about Cardiopulmonary Resuscitation: model patient information leaflet.* London: Royal College of Nursing, Resuscitation Council (UK), British Medical Association; 2008. Available at: www.resus.org.uk/pages/deccprmd.pdf (accessed 25 March 2014).
- Findlay GP, Shotton H, Kelly BA, *et al. Time to Intervene? A review of patients who underwent cardiopulmonary resuscitation as a result of an in-hospital cardiorespiratory arrest: A report by the National Confidential Enquiry into Patient Outcome and Death (2012).* London: NCEPOD; 2012. Available at: www.ncepod.org.uk/2012report1/downloads/CAP_fullreport.pdf (accessed 25 March 2014).
- General Medical Council. *Guidelines.* London: GMC; 2009. Available at: www.gmc-uk.org/guidance/ethical_guidance/end_of_life_DNACPR_decision.asp (accessed 25 March 2014).
- General Medical Council. *Treatment and Care Towards the End of Life: good practice in decision making.* Manchester: GMC; 2010. Available at: www.gmc-uk.org/static/documents/content/End_of_life.pdf (accessed 25 March 2014).
- O'Keeffe S, Redahan C, Keane P, *et al.* Age and other determinants of survival after in-hospital cardiopulmonary resuscitation. *Q J Med.* 1991; **81**(296): 1005–10.
- Raymont V, Bingley W, Buchanan A, *et al.* Prevalence of mental incapacity in medical inpatients and associated risk factors: cross-sectional study. *Lancet.* 2004; **364**(9443): 1421–7.
- Resuscitation Council (UK). *Recommended Standards for Recording "Do Not Attempt Resuscitation" (DNAR) Decisions.* London: Resuscitation Council (UK); 2009. Available at: www.resus.org.uk/pages/DNARrstd.htm (accessed 25 March 2014).
- Stewart K, Spice C, Rai GS. Where now with do not attempt resuscitation decisions? *Age Ageing.* 2003; **32**(2): 143–8.

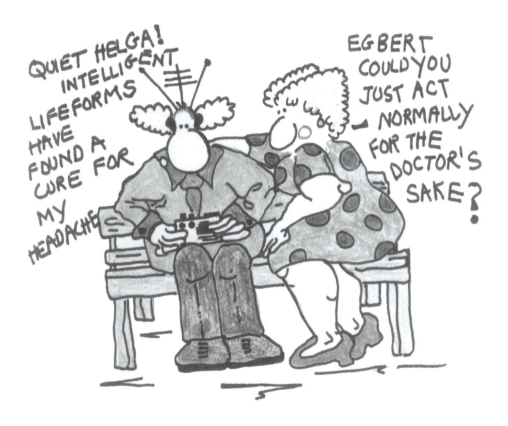

CHAPTER 7

Mental capacity and best interests

Steven Luttrell

The right of a mentally competent adult to refuse medical or any other intervention is enshrined in UK common law and reinforced by the Mental Capacity Act 2005[1] and the Human Rights Act 1998. The latter incorporates the European Convention on Human Rights into domestic law and the former codifies and adds clarity to the previously somewhat confusing common law on mental incapacity. A person may refuse treatment for reasons which are 'rational, irrational or for no reason', and the Mental Capacity Act 2005 confirms that a person should not be treated as lacking capacity because he or she makes a decision that others consider to be unwise. A doctor may be liable for assault or battery or for breach of article 8[*] of the Convention on Human Rights if they touch a person contrary to his or her wishes. If the person is mentally incapable, whether temporarily or permanently, the doctor has a duty to act in his or her best interests.

LEGAL RULES FOR ASSESSING MENTAL CAPACITY FOR MEDICAL DECISIONS

The Mental Capacity Act 2005 sets out a presumption of capacity reflecting the previous common law position – that is, that an adult has full legal capacity unless it is established that he or she does not. The burden of proof is generally on the person who is seeking to establish the lack of capacity and the decision should be made on the balance of probabilities.

Capacity must be judged in relation to the particular decision at the time that decision needs to be made. The Act clarifies that a person should not be treated as unable to make a decision until everything practicable has been done to help the person make his or her own decisions. The Mental Capacity Act 2005 Code of Practice gives guidance on a range of practicable steps that may help someone to make a decision;[2] these include minimising anxiety, waiting

---

[*] Article 8 of the Human Rights Act 1998 is the right to private and family life, and also incorporates the right to protect the physical integrity of a person.

for recovery, using support for speech or language problems and increasing the awareness of cultural, ethnic or religious factors.

Before the Mental Capacity Act 2005 came into force, the tests for assessing capacity had been determined by case law, which had led to confusion among both legal and healthcare practitioners. The definition of a person who lacks capacity is now set out under section 2 of the Act, which states that:

> a person lacks capacity in relation to a matter if at the material time he is unable to make a decision for himself in relation to the matter because of an impairment of, or a disturbance in the functioning of, the mind or brain.

Therefore, section 2 creates a two-stage test: (1) there must be an impairment or disturbance of the mind or brain and (2) this must be sufficient to render the person unable to make the decision.

The test for assessing capacity is further set out within section 3 of the Act. This is a functional test focusing on process and not on outcome. Under this a person is unable to make a decision if he or she is unable:

(i)   to understand the information relevant to the decision,
(ii) to retain that information,
(iii) to use or weigh that information as part of the process of making the decision or
(iv) to communicate his decision (whether by talking, using sign language or any other means).

The Act requires every effort to be made to provide an explanation of information relevant to the decision in a way that is appropriate to the circumstances of the person and using the most effective means of communication. It is not always necessary for the person to understand all the details; he or she must merely understand what is proposed and the possible consequences in broad terms and simple language.

The person must be able to retain the information for long enough to make the decision and the period of retention will depend on the particular decision and the amount of information required. The third criterion, relating to using or weighing information, reflects the previous common law position; see *Re MB* 1997,[3] which recognised that a range of mental health problems might prevent a person from being able to use information in a decision-making process – for example, compulsive disorders, depressive disorders. The fourth criterion, relating to communication, was intended by the Law Commission to be relevant only to a minority of people. It is not appropriate if the person is known to be incapable of deciding in which case the person would have failed one of the earlier criteria. The Code of Practice recommends that involvement of a speech and language specialist or a person with specific skills in communication may be required to assist in this aspect of the assessment.

Prior to the Mental Health Act 2005 there was a range of common law tests for assessing capacity for different types of decisions – for example, capacity for medical decisions, capacity to make a will, capacity to enter into a contract. The Act builds upon rather than contradicts these previous tests and the correct approach now is to apply the test set out in sections 2 and 3 of the Act.

For day-to-day decisions it would not be appropriate for carers or support staff to undertake detailed assessments and in these circumstances it is sufficient that the carer has a reasonable belief that the person lacks capacity for the decision in question.

ASSESSING MENTAL CAPACITY

Where consent to medical treatment or examination is required, the doctor or healthcare professional proposing the treatment must decide whether the person has capacity to consent and should record the assessment and findings in the person's healthcare record. The more serious the decision the more formal the assessment will have to be.

In cases where mental impairment is severe, the assessment may often be straightforward. However, where impairment is mild or moderate, the assessment can be difficult. In such cases the doctors should undertake a comprehensive examination of mental function, having regard to the fact that an abnormality in behaviour, language function, mood, thought, perception, insight, cognition, memory, intelligence or orientation may contribute to an inability to make a decision, thereby rendering the person mentally incapable. Evidence from other members of the multidisciplinary team, especially nursing and therapy colleagues, and also from the patient's relatives or friends, will be helpful in coming to a decision.

It is important to understand that the assessment of mental capacity is specific to the decision being undertaken. A person with borderline capacity may be able to make simple decisions concerning treatment of a straightforward nature but be unable to make a decision on a more complex issue. For some people mental capacity may fluctuate from time to time.

The assessing doctor should take the steps to minimise those reversible factors that may be affecting capacity. Some examples are as follows.

➤ Treatable medical conditions that affect mental capacity (e.g. acute confusion and depression) should be addressed, and if practicable the assessment should be delayed until capacity is optimal.

➤ Sensory impairments should be corrected if practicable.

➤ Care should be taken to choose the best location and time for the assessment.

➤ A decision should be reached as to whether the presence of a friend, relative or interpreter would be helpful.

The patient should be informed about the nature of the assessment, its implications and the process by which decisions are made. During the assessment the doctor should avoid asking leading questions.

It is important that the results of an assessment of mental capacity are clearly documented. Template systems such as the FACE Mental Capacity Assessment can provide a helpful method of ensuring that appropriate steps are taken and recorded.

MAKING DECISIONS FOR A MENTALLY INCAPABLE ADULT

Patients who are mentally incapable must be treated in their best interests. Prior to the Mental Capacity Act 2005, the principles setting out how best interests decisions should be made were reflected in the common law. The Act captures these principles in the form of a checklist set out in section 4. There is no hierarchy in the checklist and the weight to be attached to each of the factors will depend on the specific circumstances.

The Act makes it explicit that a determination of best interests must not be based merely on the person's age or appearance or any condition or aspect of the person's behaviour that might lead others to make unjustified assumptions. Mentally incapable people are to be treated no less favourably than people with capacity. The person making the decision must consider all relevant circumstances as well as the steps in the checklist. These relevant circumstances are defined as those 'of which the person making the determination is aware' and 'which it would be reasonable to regard as relevant'.

The checklist goes on to cover the following issues:
➤ recovery of capacity
➤ encouraging the person to participate
➤ non-motivation by a desire to bring about death
➤ the person's wishes feelings, beliefs and values
➤ the views of others
➤ the duties imposed by a lasting power of attorney.

The Act requires the decision-maker to consider whether it is likely that the person will at some time have capacity in relation to the matter in question, and if so, when that might be. The decision-maker should take this into account and will wish to consider whether the decision can be made at a time when it is likely that the person may have recovered capacity.

The Act also requires that even when a person does not have capacity, he or she should be both permitted and encouraged to participate, or to improve his or her participation as fully as possible, in the decision-making process or in relation to any act done to him or her.

An important aspect of the section 4 checklist relates to the wishes, feelings, beliefs and values of the individual. Under section 4 (6) the decision-maker must take into consideration:
➤ the person's past and present wishes and feelings and in particular any relevant written statements made by him when he had capacity
➤ the beliefs and values that would be likely to influence his decision if he had capacity and

➤ the other factors that he would be likely to consider if he were able to do so.

The Act also ensures that carers, family members and other relevant people are consulted on decisions affecting the person lacking capacity if it is practicable and appropriate to do so. The Code of Practice suggests that decision-makers must show that they have thought about whom to speak to, and that if it is practicable and appropriate they must speak to these people and take their views into account. The consultation is limited to two issues: what the other person considers to be in the person's best interests and whether they can provide any information about the wishes, feelings, beliefs or values of the person lacking capacity, or if prior to loosing capacity, the person had nominated another to be consulted. The requirement for consultation must be balanced against the right to confidentiality or the person lacking capacity.

In addition to other aspects of section 4, there is a specific test relating to decisions concerning the provision or withdrawal of life-sustaining treatment. The Act sets out that in determining whether a decision is in the best interests of the patient, the person making the determination must not be motivated by a desire to bring about the individual's death. The Act does not have the effect of permitting unlawful killing, and any decision about life-sustaining treatment for a person who lacks capacity must take as its starting point the assumption that it is the person's best interests for life to continue. However, there will be cases – for example, in the final stages of terminal illness – where treatment is futile or overly burdensome, where it may be in the best interests of the person to withdraw or to withhold treatment, which might incidentally shorten life.

For serious medical treatment, the Code of Practice confirms the previous case law requirements to seek a declaration from the court in cases where serious forms of medical treatment are proposed. This includes the withdrawal or withholding of life-sustaining treatment from patients in a vegetative or minimally conscious state, the proposed non-therapeutic sterilisation of a person lacking capacity or other cases involving an ethical dilemma in an untested area.

If an advance refusal of treatment is known to exist that is clear and unambiguous and is valid and applicable in the circumstances that have arisen, any health professional who knowingly provides treatment contrary to the terms of that decision may be liable to legal action for battery or assault or for breach of human rights. The Act does not protect from such liability. The applicability of advance decisions to refuse treatment is set out in sections 24–27 of the Act.

THE MENTAL HEALTH ACT 1983

The Mental Capacity Act 2005 sets out in section 28 that its decision-making powers cannot be used to give or consent to treatment for mental disorder if the treatment is regulated by the Mental Health Act 1983, part 4. Section

28 ensures that where a person lacking capacity to consent to treatment is detained under the Mental Health Act 1983, that the powers of this Act will override the decision-making powers under the Mental Capacity Act 2005. The safeguards and procedures of the Mental Health Act 1983 (as amended by the Mental Health Act 2007) cannot be avoided by reference to the Mental Capacity Act 2005.

DEPRIVATION OF LIBERTY

The deprivation of liberty safeguards were introduced into the Mental Capacity Act 2005 by the Mental Health Act 2007. They provide a framework for approving the deprivation of liberty for people who lack the capacity to consent to treatment or care either in a hospital or a care home and that in their own best interests can only be provided in circumstances that amount to a deprivation of liberty. The legislation contains detailed requirements about when and how deprivation of liberty can be authorised, setting out an assessment process that must be undertaken and arrangements for renewing and challenging decisions. Guidance on the safeguards is set out in the *Deprivation of Liberty Safeguards Code of Practice*.[4]

MEDICAL RESEARCH

Details relating to research and incapacity are set out in chapter 11 of the Code of Practice. The Act applies to research that is intrusive, involves people who have an impairment of, or disturbance in the functioning of, their mind or brain that makes them unable to decide whether or not to agree to take part in the research and is not a clinical trial covered under the Medicines for Human Use (Clinical Trials) Regulations 2004. Research covered by the Act cannot include people who lack capacity to consent unless it has the approval of an 'appropriate body'. In addition, it must follow the other requirements of the Act to consider the views of carers and other relevant people, treat the person's interests as more important that those of science and society, and respect any objections a person who lacks capacity makes during research.

In England, the 'appropriate body' must be a research ethics committee recognised by the Secretary of State. Such a body can only approve research if (1) it is linked to an impairing condition that affects the person who lacks capacity or the treatment of that condition, (2) there are reasonable grounds for believing that the research would be less effective if only people with capacity are involved and (3) the research project has made arrangements to consult carers and to follow the requirements of the Act. In addition, there are two further requirements: either (1) the research must have some chance of benefiting the person who lacks capacity and this benefit must be in proportion to the burden caused by taking part or (2) the aim of the research must be to provide knowledge about the cause of, or treatment or care of, people with the same impairing condition or a similar one.

KEY POINTS

- The right of a mentally capable adult to refuse medical or any other intervention is enshrined in UK law, and the law relating to people who are mentally incapable is set out in the Mental Capacity Act 2005.
- A person lacks capacity in relation to a matter if at the material time he or she is unable to make a decision because of an impairment of, or a disturbance in the functioning of, the mind or brain.
- A person lacks capacity if he or she is unable to understand the information relevant to the decision, retain that information, use or weigh that information as part of the process of making the decision or communicate the decision.
- If a person is mentally incapable for a particular decision, that decision must be made in that person's best interests.
- In reaching a best interests decision the decision-maker should have regard to all relevant circumstances and the various factors set out in section 4 of the Mental Capacity Act 2005.
- In reaching a best interests decision, the decision-maker should have regard to the person's wishes, feelings, beliefs and values and the views of others whom it is appropriate and practicable to consult.
- Particular requirements relating to the deprivation of liberty for a mentally incapable person are set out in the *Deprivation of Liberty Safeguards Code of Practice*.
- Particular requirements relating to the participation of a mentally incapable person in research are set out in sections 30–34 of the Mental Capacity Act 2005.

REFERENCES

1. *Mental Capacity Act 2005*. London: Department of Health; updated 2012. Available at www.justice.gov.uk/downloads/protecting-the-vulnerable/mca/mca-code-practice-0509.pdf (accessed 25 March 2014).
2. Department of Constitutional Affairs. *Mental Capacity Act 2005*. Code of Practice. London: TSO; 2008. Available at: www.justice.gov.uk/guidance/-mca-code-of-practice.htm (accessed 25 March 2014).
3. *Re MB* (medical treatment) [1997] 2 FLR 426.
4. *Deprivation of Liberty Safeguards Code of Practice to supplement the main Mental Capacity Act 2005 Code of Practice*. London: TSO; 2008.

CHAPTER 8

Testamentary capacity and the role of the physician

Gurcharan S Rai and Aza Abdulla

INTRODUCTION

Testamentary capacity is a task- and situation-specific capacity, required in law, for the individual to write and sign a will. An individual may have capacity to make a simple will but lack capacity to do other things. The person making the will (testator in the case of a man and testatrix in the case of a woman) must be over 18 years of age and be able to:

➤ understand the nature of making the will and its effects
➤ understand the extent of his or her estate – this does not mean having knowledge of the precise value of the estate but, rather, having understanding of the estate in general terms
➤ comprehend and appreciate the claims of those who might expect to benefit from the will – this includes those included in and those excluded from the will.

The testator or testatrix should not have a mental illness or disorder that influences him or her to make bequests in the will that he or she would not otherwise have included. These criteria for defining and assessing testamentary capacity are based on the judgment in the case of *Banks v Goodfellow*.[1]

In assessing testamentary capacity it is important to remember the following points.

➤ The testator or testatrix only needs to have testamentary capacity at the time he or she writes and signs the will or modifies the existing will or revokes an existing will.
➤ An individual only needs to have general understanding of the nature of a will to have testamentary capacity.
➤ In English law an individual can leave his or her belongings or wealth to

whomever he or she wishes (including a pet), as long as the individual satisfies the *Banks v Goodfellow* test.

MENTAL ILLNESS AND TESTAMENTARY CAPACITY

➤ While it is accepted that a person should not have mental illness or disorder, an individual with mental illness can still prepare a valid will.

➤ A person with fluctuating capacity can also make a will that will be regarded as valid if prepared during a lucid period.

➤ Having delusions does not invalidate the will unless the delusions have influenced the person making a particular disposition.

➤ A patient with memory impairment due to dementia may be able to concentrate to make a valid will. However, a person with severe dementia, a person receiving inpatient psychiatrist treatment or someone who is seriously ill should be formally assessed by a psychiatrist or a physician before a will is made, to confirm that he or she has testamentary capacity.

VALIDITY OF WILL

Validity of the will is decided by the court, but for a will to be valid:

➤ it must be in writing

➤ it must be signed by the person making the will – that is, the testator or testatrix

➤ the testator or testatrix's signature must be witnessed by at least two independent witnesses, and these witnesses must be present when the will is signed by the testator or testatrix.

The will is invalid if the testator or the testatrix lacks testamentary capacity at the time the will is executed.

INVOLVEMENT OF DOCTORS

Assessing testamentary capacity

Doctors may be asked to assess testamentary capacity or to give a retrospective opinion on testamentary capacity or to witness a will. Those who are asked to assess testamentary capacity should follow a process recommended by Jacoby and Steer.[2] This process is as follows:

➤ insist on a letter of instructions from the solicitor confirming that a person has consented to the examination and disclosure of the results

➤ insist on receiving full information about the patient's estate and family

➤ insist on confirmation in writing of the legal test for capacity; here it is important to remember that in civil legal matters the standard of proof is based on the balance of probabilities.

For assessment it is important that the doctor:
> assesses the patient for the presence of dementia in a standard way
> confirms that a person satisfies the *Banks v Goodfellow*[1] criteria
> records the patient's answers verbatim
> checks facts about the estate
> asks why potential beneficiaries are included or excluded from the will
> asks about and reviews previous wills
> seeks a second opinion if after the assessment there is doubt about the person's capacity.

In assessing capacity it is important that the doctor follows the guidance provided by the General Medical Council, which includes the Mental Capacity Act 2005 – that is, the doctor should presume that a person has capacity unless he or she proves otherwise thorough evidence and assessment.

Mental status and cognition assessment should include:
> assessment of mood, thought process and thought content, including delusions or hallucinations, presence or absence of paranoid ideas or suspicious beliefs
> assessment of language
> cognitive screening using the Mini-Mental State Examination (MMSE) or the clock-drawing test – here it is important to remember that the results of these tests do not provide a definitive answer as to whether the individual has or does not have testamentary capacity, but they may help the doctor support his or her conclusion.

Witnessing the will
Witnessing a will authenticates the testator or testatrix's signature and does not confirm the capacity of the individual. However, as a doctor's signature may imply that the testator or testatrix had capacity, doctors should resist acting as a witness unless they have properly assessed the person's capacity.

PERSONS WITH MENTAL INCAPACITY AND WHO HAVE NOT PREPARED A WILL
If an individual is incapable of managing his or her affairs and incapable of making a will, then the Court of Protection can be asked to draw up a statutory will, consistent with one the individual would have made. The person appointed or authorised by the court will sign with his or her name on behalf of the individual and in the presence of two witnesses. After this the will is sealed with the official seal of the Court of Protection. If the appointed/authorised individual disinherits family members, those family members may apply to the Court under the Inheritance (Provision for Family and Dependants) Act 1975 on the grounds that reasonable financial provision has not been made for them.

CASE HISTORIES

Cases 8.1 and 8.2 illustrate points made in this chapter.

CASE 8.1

An 85-year-old male patient is in hospital with delirium due to bronchopneumonia. The patient's daughter brings in a copy of a will prepared by a solicitor 2 weeks earlier and requests that a senior doctor and her friend should witness her dad signing the will.

Comment

While witnessing a will only authenticates the signature of the person who has prepared a will, it may also imply that the testator or testatrix has capacity to sign the will. Therefore, it is important that any doctor who agrees to do this assesses the testator or testatrix's capacity to prepare and sign the will and documents this assessment in his or her notes. In the case outlined here the situation is complicated by the presence of an acute illness and delirium. While individuals with delirium can and do have lucid periods, during which they may have capacity to sign a will, the doctor in this case should advise the daughter that signing of the will should be delayed until her father has fully recovered from delirium.

CASE 8.2

A solicitor acting on behalf of the daughter of an 89-year-old man, Mr A, writes a letter asking Mr A's physician, who had seen Mr A in the day hospital regularly until Mr A's death 6 months ago, to confirm that Mr A had capacity to prepare the will in 2011, 2 years before his death. In the letter of instructions the solicitor confirms that his client's brother is challenging the will.

Mr A suffered from osteoarthritis, congestive cardiac failure, chronic obstructive airways disease and Alzheimer's dementia, which was diagnosed in 2009 and for which he was prescribed donepezil with some clinical benefit. At the start of treatment his MMSE score was 24/30; by 2011 it was 18/30 and just before his death, from community-acquired pneumonia, his MMSE score was 15/30. During this period of follow-up and until his death, Mr A lived alone in his ground-floor flat. In 2011 he was independent in activities of daily living, he could prepare a small breakfast but he required help with shopping, preparation of main meals and housework, and he relied on his son to pay all his bills.

Comments

- As the patient is not alive and his testamentary capacity was not assessed or documented in 2011, the assessment can only be based on assumptions using the available clinical data.
- The doctor should only agree to provide the report if there are enough clinical

data that can be used to assess the testamentary capacity in 2011 using the *Banks v Goodfellow*[1] criteria.

- The clinical notes confirm that Mr A suffered from progressive dementia at the time of preparing and signing the will, but he was able to live independently with some help from his son in paying bills. His MMSE results in 2011 indicated he had poor short-term memory, he was disoriented to place and time, and he was unable spell the word 'world' backwards, write a sentence or draw intersecting pentagons. These results indicate that Mr A had cognitive problems, but these results by themselves do not provide sufficient evidence to make a definitive conclusion on the testamentary capacity of Mr A in 2011 – particularly as MMSE score alone does not necessarily indicate that an impairment is severe enough to affect a person's ability to instruct the drawing-up of a simple will and to then sign it.

KEY POINTS

- Testamentary capacity in law is a specific capacity to write and sign a will.
- Presence of testamentary capacity has been defined by the judgment in the case of *Banks v Goodfellow.*[1]
- Doctors asked to assess capacity should follow a process suggested by Jacoby and Steer.[2]
- The presence of delusions, delirium or dementia does not always mean that an individual lacks testamentary capacity.

REFERENCES

1. *Banks v Goodfellow* (1870) LR 5 QB 549.
2. Jacoby R, Steer P. How to assess capacity to make a will. *BMJ.* 2007; **335**(7611): 155–7.

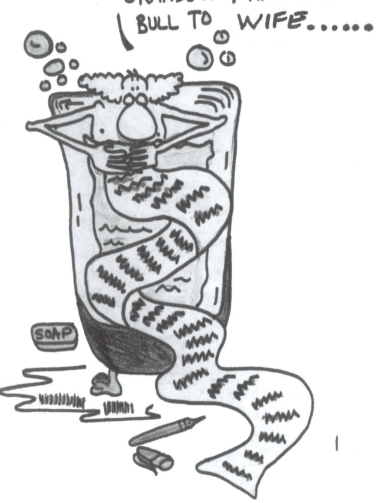

Advance decisions/advance decisions to refuse treatment

Gurcharan S Rai

INTRODUCTION

An advance decision (AD)/an advance decision to refuse treatment (ADRT), otherwise known as an advance directive or a living will,[1] is a statement of treatment preferences that indicates a person's wishes should the capacity for decision-making be lost in the future. That is, it sets out clear instruction on refusal of treatment or medical intervention or procedures. Based on the principle of autonomy, it aims to project this forward into possible future mental incapacity.

An advance consent or authorisation similarly defines a person's wishes for advance request for treatment at the time he or she loses capacity for decision-making. Unlike an AD/ADRT, these instructions are not a directive that the doctor has to comply with if it conflicts with his or her clinical judgement.

BACKGROUND

Advance directives were introduced in the United States following the case of Karen Quinlan. Karen was 21 years of age when in 1975 she developed a permanent vegetative state after taking tranquillisers and alcohol. She was maintained on a respirator with nasogastric feeding. When the Quinlan family realised there was no prospect of Karen's recovery, they requested that her life support be discontinued. There was no legal precedent for such a decision at that time, and medical opinion was firmly against the proposal. A long legal battle ensued, during which the courts involved attempted to determine what Karen's wishes would be in the circumstances then affecting her. In the event, the Supreme Court of New Jersey gave permission for Karen to be removed from the respirator. Ironically, as feeding was continued, it was not until almost 10 years later that Karen died.

Arising from this and subsequent cases, the view developed that it would be much easier to make decisions in similarly difficult circumstances if the prior wishes of the patient were known. Subsequently, advance directives have been given statutory recognition in all the states in the United States and in Canadian provinces.

A similar debate took place in the UK in the case of Tony Bland, a young man who developed a permanent vegetative state after sustaining an injury in the Hillsborough football stadium disaster. Both his doctors and his parents reached the view that after around 2 years without any improvement in his condition, artificial feeding should be discontinued. The case eventually reached the House of Lords as the highest court of appeal. The Law Lords sanctioned the withdrawal of feeding, and Tony Bland died around 4 years after being injured.

In giving judgment, a recommendation was made to the effect that Parliament should consider the issues involved. This led to the creation of the House of Lords Select Committee on Medical Ethics, which published its report in 1994.[1] In this report the term 'advance directive' is described as a 'document executed while a patient is competent, concerning his or her preferences about medical treatment in the event of becoming incompetent'. The report commended the development of ADs, but stopped short of recommending statutory legislation to support them, indicating that doctors are increasingly recognising their ethical obligations towards them, and that in any event case law is moving in the same direction.

The report makes important points concerning the implementation of an advance directive:

➤ it may express refusal of any treatment or procedure that would require the consent of the patient if competent
➤ it should not request any unlawful intervention or omission
➤ it cannot require treatment to be given that the healthcare team judge as being not clinically appropriate
➤ such directives could not be given greater legal force without depriving patients of the doctor's professional expertise and the benefit of any new treatments that may have become available since the directive was signed.

This last comment (*see* House of Lords report, paragraph 264) summarises one of the most telling objections to the value of ADs. Instead of legislation, the report recommended that the colleges and faculties of all the healthcare professions develop a code of practice to guide their members. This was taken up by the British Medical Association and resulted in the publication of *Advance Statements about Medical Treatment*.[2] The steering group was widely representative of medicine, nursing and the law. In the introduction, the code of practice stated unequivocally that the subject of ADs is quite separate from euthanasia, assisted suicide or allocation of healthcare resources. Such a distinction is clearly not shared universally – witness the support given to ADs by the Voluntary Euthanasia Society.[3] Academics, too, see the subjects as being closely related.[4]

In 2008 the General Medical Council included advice to doctors on 'advance statements' in its document on consent.[5] This is an important step, as it means that awareness of ADs and their observance is mandatory.

The Law Commission, in its report on mental incapacity,[6] recommended specific statutory recognition of advance directives, and after long consultation advance directive/refusal was included in the Mental Capacity Act 2005, which came into force in 2007.

ADVANCE DECISION/ADVANCE DECISION TO REFUSE TREATMENT AND THE LAW

Prior to the coming into force of the Mental Capacity Act 2005, in October 2007, advance decisions to refuse treatment/advance directives were legally valid under common law – the courts recognised that adults have the right to say in advance that they want to refuse treatment if they lose capacity in the future – even if this results in their death. Article 5 of the Act sets out conditions that must be met for advance refusal/advance directive to be legally valid. These conditions are as follows.

➤ An individual making or drawing up advance refusal must be an adult aged 18 or over.
➤ The person must be competent or deemed to be have capacity at the time the AD/ADRT is formulated.
➤ The AD/ADRT must specify the treatment that the person wishes to refuse, in medical and lay terms.
➤ The person can specify the circumstances in which the refusal will apply.
➤ The person making the AD/ADRT has not acted inconsistently with the terms of the refusal.
➤ The AD/ADRT must be valid and applicable. It is not valid if it is subsequently withdrawn by the person or by a lasting power of attorney (LPA) appointed by the person. It is not applicable if a person has capacity to make decision at the time of treatment or the treatment has not been specified or if unanticipated circumstances arise which are likely to have influenced the decision.
➤ The AD/ADRT dealing with life-sustaining treatment must be written, signed and witnessed and must include a statement that the decision applies even if the person's life is at risk.
➤ Refusal of non-life-sustaining treatment can be verbal.

The Mental Capacity Act 2005 only applies to England and Wales. In Scotland, the area of advance decision-making is covered by the Code of Practice issued under the Adults with Incapacity (Scotland) Act 2000, which advises that an advance decision/directive made by a competent adult should be seen as a strong indication of his or her former wishes. In Northern Ireland, common law applies, as there is no statute.

Although the Mental Capacity Act 2005 does not impose any particular requirement or constraints on the AD/ADRT form, the Mental Capacity Act 2005 Code of Practice[7] suggests that the following should be included:
> full details of the person (i.e. name, address and date of birth)
> the name and address of his or her general practitioner
> a date the document was written or withdrawn
> a clear statement on the treatment to be refused and the circumstances under which it will apply
> a statement that the ADRT should be used when he or she lacks capacity
> an individual's signature and a signature of any witness

ADs (refusals) made before the Mental Capacity Act 2005

The Act includes transitional and consequential provisions in relation to decisions made before the Act came into force. These transitional provisions accept such decisions, even though they do not comply with the specific recommendation relating to life-sustaining treatment (i.e. they do not include a statement that the decision is to apply even if life is at risk, with no signature from the person or a witness). The other conditions are as follows.
> The AD is in writing.
> The person has not withdrawn the decision at a time when he or she had capacity.
> The person does not have the capacity to give or refuse consent to the treatment in question.
> The treatment in question and the circumstances are clearly specified in the AD.
> The clinical staff have a reasonable belief that the AD/ADRT was made before 1 October 2007 and that the person has lacked capacity since that date.
> If the doctor believes that the person has had the capacity to amend his or her decision since October 2007, then the aforementioned transitional provisions will not apply.

Verbal advance decision to refuse treatment

An individual can make a verbal ADRT and professionals must follow these if they consider they exist and are valid and applicable, except if treatment is life-sustaining – here refusal must be in writing, signed and witnessed.

Advance refusal of life-prolonging treatment

Under the Mental Capacity Act 2005, advance refusal of life-sustaining treatment must be written, signed and witnessed and must include a statement that the decision applies even if the person's life is at risk.

Advance refusal of basic care

Basic or essential care – this includes provision of food and water by mouth, warmth, shelter and basic nursing care to keep the person comfortable or to reduce distress, such as the use of analgesics – cannot be included in an advance statement by an individual. However, an individual has the right to refuse these measures when offered while he or she is competent. As and when a patient becomes incompetent, he or she will still be offered basic care by healthcare professionals, for it would be unethical to deny measures to relieve suffering. Having said this, an incompetent person may still refuse to accept fluids or food by not opening his or her mouth. If healthcare professionals accept refusal as genuine, then physicians must respect this decision.

Advance decisions regarding mental treatment

There is no difference between physical or mental disorder unless a person is detained under the Mental Health Act 1983 and the treatment is being given without consent under Part 4 of the Act.

Advance decisions and lasting power of attorney

If lasting power of attorney (LPA), which gives the attorney the authority to give or refuse consent to treatment, is created after the AD/ADRT then the AD/ADRT is not valid. However, if LPA was made before the AD/ADRT then the AD/ADRT overrules the decision of an attorney under the LPA.

Protection for professionals from liability

Physicians who do not follow an AD/ADRT could face criminal prosecution or could be liable to be sued in the Civil Court. The Mental Capacity Act 2005 also provides protection to the healthcare professionals if they withhold or stop treatment because they reasonably believe that a valid and applicable AD/ADRT exists.

CONCLUSION

The ethical basis for the AD/ADRT is derived from recognition of individual autonomy. Prior to the Mental Capacity Act 2005, ADs were legally valid under common law. Article 5 of the Mental Capacity Act 2005 sets out conditions that must be met for an AD/ADRT to be legally valid. Even if the AD/ADRT is not valid and applicable it is essential to use it as strong evidence of the patient's past wishes, as part of the best interests decision-making process.

KEY POINTS

- An advance decision (AD)/an advance decision to refuse treatment (ADRT), sometimes known as a living will, is a statement of treatment preferences as an indication of a patient's wishes should his or her capacity for decision-making be lost in the future.
- An AD/ADRT had the authority of common law precedent until the Mental Capacity Act 2005, which came into force in October 2007.
- For an AD/ADRT to be valid, an individual must be an adult over 18 years of age, must be competent at the time, and must specify the treatment to be refused and the circumstances in which refusal is to apply.
- An AD/ADRT dealing with life-sustaining treatment must be written, signed and witnessed and must include a statement that the decision applies even if the person's life is at risk.
- An AD/ADRT prepared before the Mental Capacity Act 2005 came into force in 2007 is valid even if it is not signed or witnessed or if it does not contains a statement that the decision applies even if the person's life is at risk, provided the patient has remained incompetent since October 2007.
- In an emergency or where there is doubt about the existence or validity of an AD/ADRT, doctors can and should provide all the immediately necessary treatment to stabilise the medical condition or to prevent deterioration until the existence and/or validity and applicability of the AD/ADRT have been established.

CASE HISTORIES

CASE 9.1

Mrs A, who is 82 years of age, is admitted with a stroke (total middle cerebral artery infarction) and is not expected to recover. During the hospitalisation, she develops pneumonia, for which she is given intravenous antibiotics. Her son, who visits her daily, produces a copy of an advance decision, written on a pre-prepared form. This was prepared 6 months earlier, after Mrs A's sister had suffered a stroke. It is signed by Mrs A and witnessed by her general practitioner. In the statement she asserts that she would not wish to be kept alive if she suffered a severe stroke that would leave her dependent upon others for daily care. It is also stated that 'this decision applies even if my life is at risk'.

Comment

This is a valid and applicable advance statement made by an individual who, on probability, was competent at the time she prepared it. Therefore, physicians should respect it.

CASE 9.2

A 75-year-old man, Mr B, who has suffered from Parkinson's disease for 15 years and is now experiencing 'on–off' periods and difficulty with speech and swallowing despite changes to therapy recommended by the physician, is admitted with a community-acquired pneumonia and delirium. His wife, who looks after him, informs the physician that her husband is a very religious man and that he believes that life is sacred and must be preserved at all costs, even if quality seems poor. She requests that all measures, including intensive therapy unit admission, must be considered.

Comment

No one can demand treatment for him- or herself on behalf of an individual. However, views of a patient made through his or her family members or carers must be respected and used in assessing or planning treatment in his or her best interests, when he or she is no longer competent to make a decision by him- or herself. While an AD/ADRT can be verbal, a vague statement made by the patient does not form the basis of a valid AD/ADRT.

REFERENCES

1. House of Lords. *Report of the Select Committee on Medical Ethics*. London: HMSO; 1994.
2. British Medical Association. *Advance Statements about Medical Treatment*. London: BMA; 1995.
3. Davies J. *Choice in Dying*. London: Ward Lock; 1997.
4. McLean S, Britton A. *The Case for Physician-Assisted Suicide*. London: HarperCollins; 1997.
5. General Medical Council. *Consent Guidance: patients and doctors making decisions together*. Manchester: GMC; 2008. Available at: www.gmc-uk.org/guidance/ethical_guidance/consent_guidance/contents.asp (accessed 6 November 2013).
6. Law Commission. *Mental Incapacity*. Law Commission Report No. 231. London: HMSO; 1995.
7. Department for Constitutional Affairs. *Mental Capacity Act 2005 Code of Practice*. London: TSO; 2007.

FURTHER READING

- *Advance Decisions to Refuse Treatment*. www.adrtnhs.co.uk
- *Advance Decision* [form]. London: Alzheimer's Society; n.d. Available at: www.alzheimers.org.uk/advancedecisionform (accessed 25 March 2014).
- www.macmillan.org.uk/Documents/Cancerinfo/AdvanceDecisiontoRefuseTreatment Form_2013.pdf (accessed 28 March 2014).

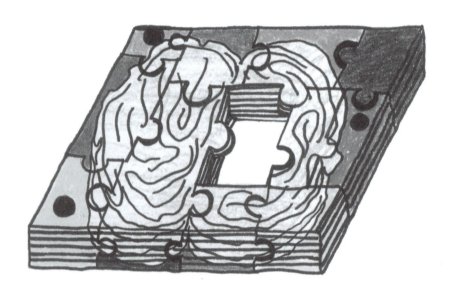

CHAPTER 10

Ethical issues in stroke management

Jonathan Birns and Gurcharan S Rai

BACKGROUND

Stroke is a common condition affecting approximately 150 000 people every year in the UK, equating to 400–500 people per year in an area served by the average district general hospital. Very few stroke survivors make a complete recovery; 12%–19% are left with speech problems, 25%–30% are unable to walk, 50% have residual weakness and 24%–53% remain dependent on carers for day-to-day activity.[1,2] Some 20% of patients will die within 1 month of the stroke and approximately 5% will be admitted to long-term residential care.

The management of stroke patients involves frequent decisions that require careful ethical consideration. In the early stages, decisions must be made against a background of uncertainty regarding the likely outcome. Later, key decisions are necessary in patients who have been left with severe disability. In addition, many stroke patients are unable to communicate their wishes with regard to treatment and placement decisions.

DIAGNOSIS

An accurate diagnosis is essential when formulating decisions about the management of a patient with an apparent stroke. A number of conditions can mimic the clinical syndrome of a stroke, including an intracranial neoplasm, subdural haematoma, intracranial abscess and hypoglycaemia. In addition, the distinction between cerebral infarction and cerebral haemorrhage cannot be accurately made on clinical grounds alone. The key investigation in establishing the diagnosis is brain imaging, via either a computed tomography scan or magnetic resonance imaging. All patients suspected of having a stroke should have brain imaging performed within 12 hours, in accordance with the Royal College of Physicians' guidelines.[3] Although these guidelines are clear, there is often an ethical issue with regard to scanning patients who may have a clinically poor prognosis or multiple disorders where the clinician believes that scanning will not change management or outcome. This may be true in some cases but there are several instances where investigations do not support initial clinical impressions and reveal an element of reversibility. Refusal to perform such a scan on the grounds of age or disability is unethical and all patients should have basic investigations, except in cases where death is imminent and to undertake investigations is likely to cause distress.

PROGNOSIS

Accurate early information regarding prognosis after stroke is crucial to enable rational decisions to be made about a patient's treatment. In a minority of cases it is clear that the patient has a very poor prognosis. For example, a patient with an extensive intracerebral bleed and impending coning or a patient with advanced dementia and a history of several previous strokes has a very poor prognosis. Early decisions to withhold possible life-prolonging measures can be made with confidence in such patients. However, the outlook for most stroke patients is much less clear. While continued assessment provides the best guide for management decisions, a number of approaches can help to provide prognostic information.

Adverse prognostic factors

A number of factors that imply a poor prognosis have been identified. These include the following:
➤ unconsciousness on admission
➤ multiple/severe co-morbidity
➤ very advanced age
➤ cognitive impairment
➤ pre-existing dependence.

Of these, a low level of consciousness on admission is the most secure indication of a poor prognosis.

STROKE SUBTYPES

Intracerebral haemorrhage confers a worse prognosis than ischaemic stroke, with haemorrhagic in-hospital and 1-year mortality rates being approximately double that of ischaemic stroke.[4] The prognosis for ischaemic stroke is also affected by the stroke subtype. The two most commonly used ischaemic stroke classification systems are the Oxfordshire Community Stroke Project[5] and TOAST (Trial of ORG 10172 in Acute Stroke Treatment) classifications.[6]

The Oxfordshire Community Stroke Project classification uses clinical localisation of the infarct topography and subdivides strokes into four groups as follows:
1. lacunar infarct – pure motor, pure sensory, sensorimotor or ataxic hemiparesis

2. total anterior circulation infarct (TACI) – higher cortical dysfunction (dysphasia or visuospatial neglect), homonymous visual field defect and hemiplegia and/or sensory deficit involving at least two areas of face, arm and leg
3. partial anterior circulation infarct – two of the three components of TACI with higher dysfunction alone or motor/sensory deficit more restricted than those classified as lacunar events
4. posterior circulation infarct – ipsilateral cranial nerve palsy with contralateral motor and/or sensory deficit, bilateral motor and/or sensory deficit, disorder of conjugate eye movement, cerebellar dysfunction or isolated homonymous visual field defect.

The TOAST classification denotes five diagnostic subgroups of ischaemic stroke, based on aetiology: large-artery atherosclerosis, cardioembolism, small-vessel occlusion (i.e. lacunar stroke), stroke of other determined aetiology and stroke of undetermined aetiology.

The prognosis for these subtypes is very different. More than 50% of patients with TACI are dead 1 year after their stroke, and the majority of those who survive a TACI will remain dependent on care to a greater or lesser degree. TACI strokes resulting from proximal occlusions of middle cerebral or internal carotid arteries may cause 'malignant' strokes that are characterised by severe neurological deficits and decreases in consciousness level that progress relentlessly to death in the majority of patients. Indeed, mortality is 80% without surgical intervention.[7] In contrast, death following a lacunar event is uncommon (less than 10% of cases at 1 year), and the majority of these patients will regain full independence. Compared with other aetiological subtypes, patients with stroke due to large-artery atherosclerosis are three times as likely to have early recurrence within 1 month,[8] and patients with stroke due to cardioembolism or undetermined aetiology have a worse prognosis in terms of disability and mortality.[9]

SCORING SCALES

A number of scoring systems have been developed in order to predict outcome. The most widely used acute stroke scoring system is the National Institutes of Health Stroke Scale that may confer an accurate probability of recovery if used in the first week (*see* Figure 10.1).[10] A score higher than 16 implies a poor prognosis, while one below 6 implies a good prognosis.

Therefore a number of factors may be taken into account when attempting to provide a patient and his or her family with accurate information about the likelihood of recovery. An accurate estimate of a patient's chances of improvement also provides a framework to aid decision-making. However, it must be remembered that the presentation in an individual patient is key, and that patients who at face value would appear to have a poor prognosis may do surprisingly well.

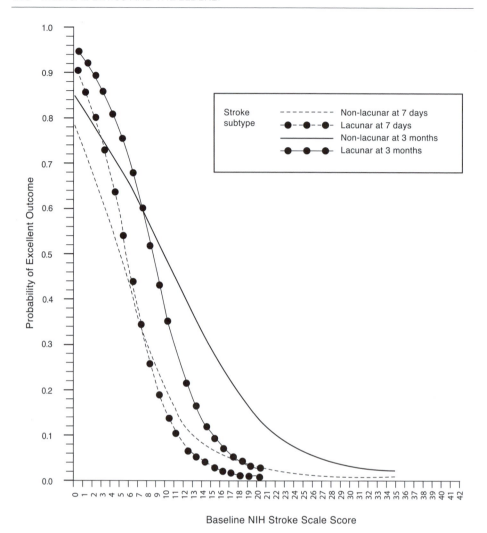

FIGURE 10.1 Probability of an excellent outcome from stroke by National Institutes of Health (NIH) Stroke Scale score[10]

CASE 10.1

A previously well 69-year-old man was admitted with a dense left hemiplegia. He was semi-conscious, with a Glasgow Coma Scale (GCS) score of 9. A computed tomography scan showed a large basal ganglia bleed with mass effect. Despite the bleed and the low GCS score, it was felt that he might do well once the haematoma had resolved. Aggressive supportive treatment including nasogastric feeding and antibiotics was used. The patient's GCS score rose to 15, 3 weeks after admission, and after rehabilitation he was discharged home, requiring only a small amount of help with personal care.

DRUG TREATMENT

Thrombolysis with recombinant tissue plasminogen activator is an accepted form of treatment for acute ischaemic stroke within 4½ hours of stroke onset in selected patients.[3,11,12] However, national clinical guidelines advise that thrombolysis should only be administered by personnel trained in its use in a centre equipped to investigate and monitor patients appropriately.[3] Non-administration of thrombolysis to a suitable patient may be regarded by some clinicians as being unethical and clinical strategies have been developed to ensure that all stroke patients have access to specialist hyper-acute stroke care.[11,13]

NUTRITION AND HYDRATION

Approximately 45% of stroke patients will have some degree of dysphagia and associated aspiration immediately after their stroke. This will resolve in over 90% of cases during the next 3 months. Many of these patients will be able to take a soft diet, but some will have a severe degree of dysphagia that precludes oral feeding and will require an alternative route to be found.

The provision of nutrition and hydration has been regarded as different to the provision of medical treatments. The law regards nutrition and hydration as a basic human right. However, the issue is clouded because both of the means used to provide nutrition and hydration in dysphagic stroke patients (nasogastric tubes and intravenous cannulae) fall under the heading of 'medical interventions'. Thus it can be argued that such treatments (as with any medical treatment) can be provided or withheld at the discretion of the treating medical team, provided decisions are based after full assessment of the individual's case. Decisions concerning nutrition are perceived as being more complex than concerning hydration because the means used to provide nutrition (nasogastric tubes) is deemed more uncomfortable (and thus less acceptable) than the means used to provide hydration. To complicate matters further, there is a dearth of evidence to guide decisions concerning nutrition, particularly the timing of initiation of enteral feeding. While the FOOD trial demonstrated that early tube feeding may reduce the risk of dying after stroke, the results suggested that improved survival may be at the expense of increasing the chances of poor outcome.[14]

It is generally accepted that withholding nutrition and hydration from a stroke patient in the early stages is unethical unless the prognosis is clearly hopeless. Usual practice is to commence nasogastric feeding within 24 hours of admission. Very often patients pull out nasogastric tubes with their good hand, increasing the probability of complications associated with repeated tube insertion. There are also ethical issues surrounding the use of restraint to prevent such patients from dislodging nasogastric tubes (*see* Chapter 15, 'The lawful use of restraints'). Gastrostomy tubes provide a more secure route for feeding as well as a more reliable supply of nutrition. However, at present there is no evidence to support the immediate use of gastrostomy tubes, and their insertion requires a surgical procedure and exposes the patient to potential complications.

Withdrawal of feeding

Withdrawal of nutrition at a later date in a patient who has not improved and who remains very disabled may be an appropriate action. If one regards nutrition via tube feeding as a medical intervention, then according to the medical model, if the indication for such an intervention no longer exists, that intervention can be withdrawn. However, before making a decision on withdrawal of nutrition it is recommended that doctors:

➤ consult the patient if he or she has the capacity to participate in the discussion, unless death is imminent and discussion with the patient about benefits, burdens and risks will not be appropriate;
➤ consult all members of the healthcare team and those close to the patient.

In some cases, it may be judicious to seek a second expert opinion from a senior clinician who has experience of the patient's condition but is not involved in the patient's care. If significant conflicts arise between members of the healthcare team, or between the healthcare team and relatives/carers, about whether artificial nutrition should be provided, legal advice should be sought.

Withdrawal of feeding is an emotive subject but discussions of this nature may be made much easier if there is appropriate counselling of the relatives before feeding is commenced. It may remain very difficult to withdraw nutrition in a conscious patient because of fears about the symptomatic effects of lack of nutrition and, in practice, nutrition is often continued as a palliative intervention, long after there is any hope of a meaningful recovery.

CHEST INFECTION AND ANTIBIOTICS

The high incidence of dysphagia coupled with other factors – such as reduced mobility, undernutrition and exposure to hospital pathogens – means that chest infection (and, more specifically, pneumonia) is a common problem in patients with acute stroke. In a severely disabled stroke patient, clinicians are often faced with the difficult decision of whether to treat such an infection, or whether it is kinder to withhold medication and allow nature to take its course. The latter decision is difficult to support in the early stages of stroke treatment in view of the problems discussed earlier about initial post-stroke prognostic judgements. One may also note that the administration of intravenous antibiotics is acceptable and generally not distressing to the patient and his or her relatives, even allowing for the potential side effects of such agents. Thus, it is common practice (and ethically sound) to treat such infections in the early stages of stroke management. The situation may be very different if the same patient with the same severe degree of disability develops pneumonia 3 months later. By this stage, the lack of potential for further recovery is clear and a decision to withhold treatment is ethically and morally supportable.

RESUSCITATION ORDERS

Much controversy exists over the rationale behind the allocation of 'do not attempt resuscitation' (DNAR) orders. The tendency in stroke patients (more than for most other conditions in acute medicine) is for a high proportion of patients to be allocated a DNAR order.

Medically, there are sound reasons why DNAR orders may be appropriate in stroke patients, even in the acute setting. Stroke patients who undergo cardiopulmonary resuscitation (CPR) have been shown to have a reduced chance of survival[15] and concern has been raised about the detrimental effects of the resuscitation process on cerebral perfusion in a patient who is already suffering a degree of brain injury. It is feared that a stroke patient who survives a resuscitation effort will be left with a more severe degree of brain injury and thus greater disability. Furthermore, concern exists over the ability of a stroke patient to survive and be successfully weaned from mechanical ventilation subsequent to initially successful CPR. However, studies of CPR outcome in hospital have often excluded large numbers of stroke patients (because of the frequency with which they are allocated DNAR orders) and thus may not provide a true picture of the potential for survival among such patients. It must also be remembered that stroke patients often have coexistent ischaemic heart disease, which has the potential to cause transient, treatable arrhythmia (e.g. ventricular fibrillation). Further, many stroke patients, particularly those with lacunar infarcts, have a very good prognosis, and issuing such a patient with a DNAR order solely because he or she has had a stroke is unlikely to be defensible.

Guidelines issued by the British Medical Association, the Resuscitation Council (UK) and the Royal College of Nursing[16] make the following recommendations.

➤ If a doctor believes that CPR will not restart the heart and maintain breathing, it should not be offered or attempted.
➤ CPR need not be offered when a patient is in the final stages of an incurable illness and death.
➤ It is lawful to withhold CPR on the basis that it would not be in the best interests of the patient. Neither the patient, nor his or her family or carers can demand CPR that is clinically inappropriate.
➤ If CPR may be successful in restarting the patient's heart and maintaining breathing for a sustained period, the benefits must be weighed against potential burdens and harms to the patient. However, this decision should consider the patient's wishes and beliefs if he or she has capacity. If such a patient chooses or wants to delay death, even for a very short period, this wish should be taken seriously under the Human Rights Act 1998.
➤ In those who lack capacity, decision-making must be based in the patient's best interests in line with the Mental Capacity Act 2005.

Finally, it must be understood that a decision not to resuscitate is not the same as a decision not to treat and that issues concerning the administration of antibiotics and so forth are quite separate.

CASE 10.2

A 58-year-old man suffered a large intracerebral bleed with a resulting dense hemiplegia, hemianopia and dysphasia. Three months after his stroke, he was transferred to another hospital for further management. No clear decision regarding resuscitation status had been made at the first hospital. A series of difficult interviews were held with the patient's family. The medical staff made clear their view that a DNAR order should be issued. The family was initially opposed to this, as they felt that such a decision would be tantamount to killing their relative. However, after many discussions they agreed with the medical viewpoint and the DNAR order was issued.

PLACEMENT

A common problem in the later stages of stroke management concerns issues about the patient's destination on discharge from hospital. Two basic rules are unavoidable. The patient should be discharged to where he or she wishes to go if at all possible, and although this may not always be possible, no patient should be forcibly discharged to somewhere he or she does not wish to go. The patient's right to self-determination as enshrined in law requires these conditions to be met. Problems arise in those patients who refuse to accept the danger of returning to an unsuitable environment. The law is quite clear about this situation – a mentally competent adult has the right to do what he or she wishes, and the clinician must accede to this.

In cases where concerns exist about the patient's decision-making ability, the patient's mental capacity should be assessed formally, in line with the Mental Capacity Act 2005.[17] The Act states that a person is unable to make a decision for him- or herself if he or she is unable to:
➤ understand the information relevant to the decision
➤ retain that information
➤ use or weigh that information as part of the process of making the decision
➤ communicate his or her decision (whether by talking, using sign language or any other means).

It should be remembered that a person must be assumed to have capacity unless it is established that he or she lacks capacity and that a person is not to be treated as unable to make a decision unless all practicable steps to help him or her to do so have been taken without success. This is particularly important in stroke patients with dysphasia whose communicative ability is limited. Skilled patient assessment by healthcare professionals, including speech and language therapists, may establish that the patient can communicate his or her wishes in some way.[18] In such cases, decisions about placement should be delayed until appropriate specialist assessments have been undertaken. It should also be borne in mind that an act done, or decision made, under the

Mental Capacity Act 2005 for or on behalf of a person who lacks capacity must be done, or made, in his or her best interests.[17]

If a patient lacks capacity for decisions pertaining to discharge, the clinical team must first enquire if, under a lasting power of attorney, the patient has appointed another person to make decisions about the patient's personal welfare, property and affairs.[17] If no such attorney has been appointed, the healthcare team should act in the patient's best interests, taking into account the patient's past and present expressed wishes, beliefs and values and the views of his or her family, friends and carers. The plans made by the healthcare team should be discussed with the patient's family and/or friends to seek their agreement. If the family and/or friends are not in agreement with the care plan or if there is no individual (such as a family member, friend, carer or neighbour) who can act as an advocate, the healthcare team should seek formal advocacy from an independent mental capacity advocate to ensure that the proposed management and discharge planning is in the best interests of the patient.

CASE 10.3

A 78-year-old gentleman who had previously lived alone suffered a left middle cerebral artery territory stroke, resulting in right-sided neurologic deficits and dysphasia and a dependency on nursing staff for personal care. The members of the healthcare team responsible for his rehabilitation and disability management were in agreement that it would not be safe for this gentleman to return home and that it would be in his best interests to be discharged to a care home. He was assessed as lacking capacity for making decisions about discharge from hospital and had no relatives or friends who could act as an advocate for him. An independent mental capacity advocate was involved to facilitate discharge decisions and they were in agreement with the plan for his transfer to a care home.

Driving after stroke

Legally, patients who have suffered a stroke or transient ischaemic attack should not drive for a month after the event. The patient should be advised to inform the Driver and Vehicle Licensing Agency (DVLA) and his or her insurance company. After a month, patients may resume driving if this is deemed safe by their clinician. In cases of doubt, an assessment at a Driver Assessment Unit may provide confirmation of a patient's degree of fitness to drive.

Some manifestations of stroke (e.g. homonymous hemianopia) disqualify the patient from driving. The clinician is negligent if he or she does not inform the patient of this fact, and, indeed, this same clinician may be held legally liable should an accident ensue. If a patient who is unfit to drive is known to be continuing to drive and will not inform the DVLA, the clinician can break confidentiality and inform the DVLA him- or herself. In these circumstances, the clinician's responsibility to society outweighs his or her responsibility to maintain confidentiality.

KEY POINTS

- Only in a very small minority of stroke patients is it possible to state that their prognosis is virtually hopeless within the first few days.
- All patients other than those with no chance of recovery should receive nutrition and hydration and should have brain imaging performed.
- Withdrawal of treatment may be justified in a patient in whom a poor prognosis has become clearer with the passage of time.
- Other potentially life-saving treatments (e.g. antibiotics) should not be withheld while the prognosis is uncertain.
- It is acceptable to issue a DNAR order while continuing all other treatments.
- It is unacceptable to issue a DNAR order to a patient solely because he or she has had a stroke.
- The clinician is ethically and legally justified in deciding treatments that are in the patient's best interests for those who cannot express their wishes, provided the clinician followed the guidance included in the Mental Capacity Act 2005.
- Communication with patients and relatives at all stages is the best way to ensure acceptability of decisions.

REFERENCES

1. Sacco RL. Risk factors, outcomes, and stroke subtypes for ischemic stroke. *Neurology*. 1997; **49**(5 Suppl. 4): S39–44.
2. Thom T, Haase N, Rosamond W, *et al.* Heart disease and stroke statistics – 2006 update: a report from the American Heart Association Statistics Committee and Stroke Statistics Subcommittee. *Circulation*. 2006 Feb 14; **113**(6): e85–151. Epub 2006 Jan 11.
3. Royal College of Physicians. *National Clinical Guidelines for Stroke*. London: RCP; 2012.
4. Christensen MC, Munro V. Ischemic stroke and intracerebral hemorrhage: the latest evidence on mortality, readmissions and hospital costs from Scotland. *Neuroepidemiology*. 2008; **30**(4): 239–46.
5. Bamford J, Sandercock P, Dennis M, *et al.* Classification and natural history of clinically identifiable subtypes of cerebral infarction. *Lancet*. 1991; **337**(8756): 1521–6.
6. Adams HP Jr, Bendixen BH, Kappelle LJ, *et al.* Classification of subtype of acute ischemic stroke. Definitions for use in a multicenter clinical trial. TOAST. Trial of Org 10172 in Acute Stroke Treatment. *Stroke*. 1993; **24**(1): 35–41.
7. Manawadu D. Malignant stroke syndrome. In: Kalra L, Wolfe C, Rudd A, editors. *A Practical Guide to Comprehensive Stroke Care*. World Scientific Publishing; 2010. pp. 185–224.
8. Lovett JK, Coull AJ, Rothwell PM. Early risk of recurrence by subtype of ischemic stroke in population-based incidence studies. *Neurology*. 2004; **62**(4): 569–73.
9. Pinto A, Tuttolomondo A, Di Raimondo D, *et al.* Risk factors profile and clinical

outcome of ischemic stroke patients admitted in a Department of Internal Medicine and classified by TOAST classification. *Int Angiol.* 2006; **25**(3): 261–7.

10. Adams HP Jr, Davis PH, Leira EC, *et al.* Baseline NIH Stroke Scale score strongly predicts outcome after stroke: a report of the Trial of Org 10172 in Acute Stroke Treatment (TOAST). *Neurology.* 1999; **53**(1): 126–31.

11. Birns J, Kalra L. Thrombolytic therapy for stroke. *Therapy.* 2009; **6**(5): 733–45.

12. Lees KR, Bluhmki E, von Kummer R, et al. Time to treatment with intravenous alteplase and outcome in stroke: an updated pooled analysis of ECASS, ATLANTIS, NINDS, and EPITHET trials. *Lancet.* 2010; **375**(9727): 1695–703.

13. Department of Health. *National Stroke Strategy.* London: DH; 2007.

14. Dennis MS, Lewis SC, Warlow C; FOOD Trial Collaboration. Effect of timing and method of enteral tube feeding for dysphagic stroke patients (FOOD): a multicentre randomised controlled trial. *Lancet.* 2005; **365**(9461): 764–72.

15. De Vos R, Koster R, De Haan RJ, *et al.* In-hospital cardiopulmonary resuscitation: pre-arrest morbidity and outcome. *Arch Intern Med.* 1999; **159**(8): 845–50.

16. British Medical Association. *Decisions Relating to Cardiopulmonary Resuscitation. A joint statement from the British Medical Association, the Resuscitation Council (UK) and the Royal College of Nursing.* London: BMA; 2007.

17. *Mental Capacity Act 2005.* London: Office of Public Sector Information. Available at: www.legislation.gov.uk/ukpga/2005/9/contents (accessed 25 March 2014).

18. Carrington S, Birns J. Establishing capacity in a patient with incomplete locked-in syndrome. *Progress in Neurology and Psychiatry.* 2012; **16**(6): 18–20.

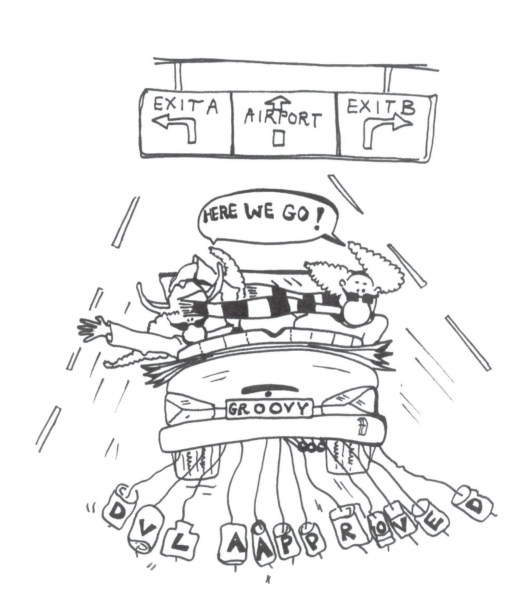

CHAPTER 11

Ethics of driving assessment in dementia: care, competence and communication

Desmond O'Neill and David Robinson

BACKGROUND

'We are bringing you to Dr O'Neill so that he can put you in a nursing home' would be a poor advertisement for a prospective patient with age-related disease about to attend a geriatric medicine clinic. The reasons for the unease generated by this phrase for both patients and practitioners are a useful guide to some of the issues related to ethics and driving. Both groups would be much happier with a formula along the lines of 'We are bringing you to Dr O'Neill to maximise your chances of staying at home. Of course, at some stage you may no longer be able to manage at home, and we may need to consider other options in the future.'

So what is the difference? The second formula:

➤ puts the needs and wishes of the patient to the fore, rather than those of the carer or society

➤ promotes the concept of geriatric medicine as enabling rather than disabling

➤ recognises a style of practice consistent with the World Health Organization[1] and United Nations[2] guidelines that promote due attention to prevention, health gain, health maintenance and palliation

➤ recognises the role of geriatric medicine in changing a societal mindset towards disabling conditions of later life. Prior to the pioneering work of Marjory Warren, the response of society was a prosthetic one, reinforcing disability by premature admission to residential care. The key advance of geriatric medicine was to bring a diagnostic and therapeutic emphasis to the care of older people.

The contextual setting of the ethics of driving often seems to neglect the simple principles of care, competence and communication: 'care' in the sense of the appropriate focus of the practitioner–patient interaction, 'competence' in the sense of knowing not only the literature of assessment and remediation but also the extent of societal ageism, and 'communication' in the sense of understanding the skills needed to move from a primary focus on health gain to one of palliation.[3] The primary ethos still appears to be 'We are bringing you to Dr O'Neill so that he can stop your driving' rather than 'We are bringing you to Dr O'Neill to maximise your changes of maintaining your mobility and transportation. Of course, at some stage you may no longer be able to drive, and we may need to consider other options in the future'. The literature in this area is a gloomy testament to the underdeveloped nature of the debate. The vast majority of the papers on MEDLINE still focus on who should not drive, rather than considering the health implications of inadequate access to transport.

RESEARCH AND PUBLIC HEALTH ETHICS

The mis-emphasis, shared also with older drivers, probably arises from a number of sources as outlined in a recent review.[4] In the context of research these include inadequate gerontological input into research groups, the distorting influence of funding sources whose primary emphasis is safety rather than mobility, and conflicts of interest of those promoting commercial driver screening methodologies of dubious value. An ethical imperative for such researchers and public health professionals is to become aware of the due proportionality of mobility and safety, and the importance of maintaining the balance in later life.

This will require a major change of attitude in public health: it is notable that the chapter on transport in one of the key texts of public health, Marmot and Wilkinson's otherwise excellent *Social Determinants of Health*,[5] makes for grim reading – accidents, pollution and the impact of cars on exercise, and no mention on how lack of access to transport is associated with impaired health and social inclusion, an emerging research issue.[6] It is encouraging that a forum has developed at the US Transportation Research Board to tease out a broader perspective on health and transport (www.trbhealth.org).

The challenge to geriatricians and gerontologists in relation to age-related disease and driving is to realign the context of mobility and risk. Some progress has already been made in this regard – the major impact of age-related disease is to curtail mobility.[7] A more measured sense of perspective has allowed a precious emphasis on risk to be reviewed – it is clear that older drivers are one of the safest groups of drivers on the road. A 2001 Organisation for Economic Co-operation and Development report,[8] entitled *Ageing and Transport*, has re-emphasised that the main public health concerns of ageing and driving are, first, reduced mobility and, second, the hazard of increased frailty in an automotive and traffic environment that is not tailored to the needs of older people. Although older people as a group are the safest category of drivers on the road, the Organisation for Economic Co-operation and Development pointed out the need for wider diffusion of assessment routines for clinicians dealing with drivers with known age-related disease.

DRIVING: A RIGHT AND A PRIVILEGE

Certain publications on driving assert that the possession of a driving licence is a privilege, but in reality it is probably both a right and a privilege. All of our societies place a higher premium on mobility than on safety. If safety were the first priority, then the speed limit would be 20 miles per hour and car engines would be fitted with governors to prevent them exceeding this speed. The right to drive carries an implicit understanding of bearing a risk that is within certain societal norms. At all levels, older drivers as a group bear a risk that is low. A false argument is sometimes presented that their accident rate per mile travelled is high. This is false for two reasons: first, because they drive a lower mileage, their annual risk remains low; second, low mileage is intrinsically risky. If older and younger drivers are controlled for low mileage, their apparent increased risk disappears.[9,10]

These positive aspects of ageing are often underappreciated, and the literature on ageing and mobility could benefit from a greater emphasis on the beneficial aspects of ageing.[4] These include wisdom, strategic thinking and less risk-taking. Even within the small proportion of crashes caused by drivers in this age group, the contribution of chronic disease to the crash risk is modest.[11] Indeed, in groups of drivers with conditions relevant to medical fitness to drive, those over 75 years of age (who had the highest level of multi-morbidity) had the lowest annual crash rate of all age groups.[12] The safety record of older drivers in the face of these odds points to superior strategic and tactical skills. If skills were more widely applied, these qualities could enhance mobility and safety for all age groups.

ETHICAL HAZARDS IN CLINICAL SETTINGS

The ethical risks to practitioners in clinical practice are failure to consider driving as a part of their patient's functional status, a tendency to police rather than to enable, failure to refer appropriately for competence assessment, inappropriate disclosure of information, and a failure to facilitate alternative transportation. The most striking example of failure to consider driving as a health-related issue comes from a study at a syncope clinic where referring physicians failed to alert many drivers (including lorry drivers!) that they should stop driving until assessment and treatment were concluded.[13] There is some evidence that this agnosia is waning with time, although knowledge remains patchy.[14]

Against this background it is important to remember the primary duties and ethical responsibilities of the physician. First, to do no harm implies avoiding the damage to lifestyle, self-esteem and subsequently health that restrictions on driving may incur. For this reason we prefer to emphasise the empowering role of the physician – there is already much emphasis in the literature on limiting a patient's ability to drive. It is a physician's duty to promote the well-being of his or her patient, and it is important to remind ourselves that our role should be to enable patients to fulfil their potential, rather than to restrict it. Respecting patients' autonomy should enable us to allow patients to accept their own risk, but all too often they are not given this choice.

There has been a modest but significant increase in the literature on disease and driving. Some of this is original research and some represents a synthesis of prevailing wisdom. In many areas, physicians have more information than they did 10 years ago. For example, with implantable cardiac defibrillators we know that the risk of crashes due to the defibrillator is low,[15] and we can predict those most at risk for syncope.[16] For cataracts, we know that older drivers with cataract experience a restriction in their driving ability and a decrease in their safety on the road.[17] We also know that surgical intervention can benefit older patients in terms of subjectively improved visual function and distance estimation while driving.[18] Such intervention translates to improved safety on the road.[19] For arthritis, while over half of patients affected report some difficulty driving,[20] we know not only that doctors fail to inquire about the impact of arthritis on mobility[21] but also that a rehabilitative intervention programme can improve driving ease.[22] For diabetes, we have increasing evidence that the condition on its own has little or no effect on crash risk among older drivers without a history of crashes.[23]

ASSESSMENT

The assessment of patients' driving ability therefore requires certain minimum standards in order to assess fairly both ability to drive and risk to others. This involves remaining up to date with best practice, being aware of local legislation, and remaining cognisant of the massive impact that we have on a person's lifestyle. The competence required is that patients will have the most accurate assessment possible of their driving abilities. Schemata exist for the preliminary work in this area for physicians in primary care (e.g. the UK,[24] Australia,[25] Canada[26] and the United States[27]), and a comprehensive review of assessment of fitness to drive with dementia was published in 2007.[28]

Just as not all chest pains arise from pulmonary emboli, clinicians need to have access to appropriate specialist expertise and technology to exclude the diagnosis in such cases. While not needed for all age-related conditions, routine access to specialist driving assessment is needed for all those with established dementia driving, and needs to be repeated at regular intervals. This may be facilitated at a specialist centre, the components of which are medicine, occupational therapy, sometimes neuropsychology and specialist driving assessors. A first effort may be made with a suitably trained occupational therapist – this profession is notable for upskilling in driving assessment in Australia, Canada and the United States. If this assessment is inconclusive, an on-road assessment is advisable for all of those with dementia. In the UK, such assessments are available from the Forum of Mobility Centres (www.mobility-centres.org.uk). In the United States, the Association for Driver Rehabilitation Specialists (www.driver-ed.org) can provide a list of suitably qualified driving assessors. It is important to emphasise to the patient that this test is not the driving test used for learner drivers but, rather, it is an assessment designed to gain insight into the capabilities and difficulties of the driver.

THERAPEUTIC MANAGEMENT AND RISK ASSESSMENT

It is the placing of driving issues in an appropriate therapeutic context that is perhaps the most important task – non-clinician bioethicists thrive on the artificial heightening of potential conflict inherent in such situations. Rather than focusing on the difficult issue of patients who present late with impaired ability and insight, we need to recognise that the assessment of dementia provides the potential for a range of interventions, one of the most important of which is the establishment of a framework for advance planning in a progressive disease.

Just as this is commonly recognised for such practical matters as lasting power of attorney in many jurisdictions, so too we need to start a process that encompasses an assessment and a commitment to maximising mobility, but also a process of awareness-raising for the patient and his or her carers that the progression of the disease will inevitably result in a loss of driving capacity. This latter component has been termed a Ulysses contract (after the hero who made his crew tie him to the mast of the ship on the condition that they did not heed his entreaties to be released when seduced by the song of the Sirens).[29]

Developing this process incorporates some new stances in dementia care. In particular, disclosure of the diagnosis in at least general terms – the patient who drives needs to be told that he or she has a memory problem that is likely to progress and hamper his or her driving abilities. In general, carers are fearful of diagnosis disclosure[30] but older people seem to want to be told if they have this illness.[31] There is also evidence that such a process may facilitate driver cessation by enhancing a therapeutic dimension to disease diagnosis and advance planning.[32] It forms the basis of a useful patient and carer brochure from the Hartford Foundation, which is also available online.[33]

The commitment to maximising mobility must focus first on as accurate an assessment of the patient's driving abilities as possible, and second on exploring and planning alternative options for a future when driving is no longer possible. It is the promise of an attempt to maximise mobility that is the key to this transaction. If this is not a central component, we are faced with a dual ethical hazard. In the first instance, the therapeutic role of medicine is subjugated to an approach, which inverts the standard of mobility/safety ratio to which we are all entitled. A further concern is that people with dementia may avoid assessment of the illness early in its course out of fear of unreasonable restriction of their mobility. As early diagnosis, treatment and management are considered to be desirable, this would be an unwelcome development.

The very act of highlighting the potential for compromised driving ability may have a therapeutic benefit, promoting increased vigilance on the part of the patient and carers about the fact that their social contract for driving privileges is not the same as that of the general public. Some support is given to this concept by the success of restricted licensing for people with medical illnesses in the state of Utah.[34] Although some of the effect might be due to the restrictions (avoidance of motorways and night-time driving), it is also possible that the very act of labelling these drivers may heighten their self-awareness.

The ethical component of risk is the onus on the physician to ensure that this has been assessed in the most accurate and professional manner possible. The greatest risk is to fail to refer the patient on for full assessment, perhaps on the basis that such expertise is geographically distant. Bear in mind that we would not let this deter us from arranging specialist neuroradiology for a suspected subdural haematoma or a ventilation/perfusion scan for a possible pulmonary embolus. We should apply similar criteria to the need for specialised assessments for impaired older drivers, particularly in view of the potential risk to other road users.

A key ethical imperative of assessment is factoring in alternative transportation inasmuch as it is possible. This is a major problem: once they reach the age of 70, it is estimated that older women may spend 10 years of their remaining 21 years without driving, and men may spend 7 of their remaining 18 years without driving.[35] While hugely impressive models of alternative transportation have been developed, such as ITNAmerica (www.itnamerica. org),[36] for those without friends, neighbours or relatives to provide transportation,[37] some knowledge of local sources of alternative transportation is vital.[38] Public transport generally will not do, as the disabilities that prompt driving cessation generally preclude use of public transport.

DISCLOSURE AND CONFIDENTIALITY

In general, the welfarist role of the physician extends to reminding the patient that most insurance companies require disclosure by the driver of 'illnesses relevant to driving' when they arise. Two issues arise. First, the medical advisers of the insurance companies may not make calculations of insurance rates (or continued insurance) on the basis of reason and evidence, but rather on ageist grounds and prejudice against disability. We may be unwittingly exposing the patient to this prejudice, although I am reassured in my own practice that the insurance companies have not put an extra loading on drivers with dementia who have declared their illness and who are undertaking appropriate regular assessments.[4] The answer to this lies in continued advocacy by professional groups at a societal level as well as support by the physician in individual cases if the assessment supports preserved driving skills.

A second issue is whether it is sufficient to recommend disclosure to someone who will not remember this advice. However, the physician's role is primarily to ensure safe mobility, and in general it is reasonable to assume that removal of insurance cover is a secondary matter in such cases. It is reasonable to share the disclosure of information with the carers.

The actual process of breaking confidentiality in the event of evidence of hazard to other members of the public is almost universally supported by most codes of medical practice. However, the question of to whom this should be reported poses some ethical challenges. The traditional route of reporting to driver licensing authorities (the Division of Motor Vehicles[39] in the United States, and the Driver and Vehicle Licensing Agency in the UK) may have relatively little benefit, as removal of a driving licence is likely to have little impact on many drivers whose insight into deteriorating driving skills is poor. It is important that this disclosure has some likelihood of impact and results in the least traumatic removal of the compromised older driver from the road. In such instances, the family may be able to intervene in terms of disabling the car and providing alternative modes of transport. In our own experience, we rarely have to invoke official intervention, but find that a personal communication with a senior police officer in the patient's locality may result in a sensitive visit to the patient and cessation of driving.

We may have laid too much emphasis in the literature on medical fitness to drive guidelines on the role and responsibility of the doctor, and not enough on the responsibilities of drivers and other citizens, and have thereby perhaps over-medicalised the response. At the point where concerns arise over continued driving by a driver with dementia and it is clear that the patient's driving habits are dangerous, it is a misguided kindness to deal with dangerous driving as an issue to be approached in terms of diagnosis and treatment of the underlying cause. As dangerous driving represents a hazard to the driver and other road users and is a statutory offence, it should be reported to the police in the first instance.

This approach can lift a weight off the doctor's shoulders, as not uncommonly a relative will ask the doctor to do something about dangerous driving that the relative has witnessed in a driver with dementia. This is second-hand information, and the doctor should remind the relative that he or she has a citizen's duty to report the dangerous driving to the police: the medical aspects can be dealt with subsequently.

Mandatory reporting presents a different ethical challenge. It is increasingly clear that it does not confer safety benefits and is likely to distort patient–doctor relationships,[40,41] and the profession should resist the introduction of such schemes and fight against the maintenance of established schemes.[42] For individual practitioners in jurisdictions where such regulations exist, a twin-track approach is probably necessary, involving professional advocacy with lawmakers, and a considered approach as to whether disclosure is in the patient's best interests on a case-by-case basis. If the physician is confident that the state or province has a mechanism for fair assessment and an enlightened approach to maintaining mobility, compliance is not difficult. If the assessment is cursory and aimed at unduly restricting mobility, physicians may be faced with a problem that is recognised with other laws, which may put patients' welfare at risk, and where professional obligations may require non-compliance with an unfair law.

CONCLUSION

The inclusion of driver assessment in clinical practice represents a new departure for the disciplines of applied ethics and ageing studies. It presents both challenges and opportunities, and involves not only clinicians but also researchers and public health professionals in ensuring that our practice represents a judicious balance between beneficence and non-maleficence, while at the same time keeping a firm perspective on the major issue, which is impaired mobility. The critical elements of care, competence and communication are the fundamentals of clinical practice that help to illuminate and clarify this equilibrium.

KEY LEGAL POINTS

- In most countries, the legal obligation to disclose medical conditions that may impair driving lies with the driver.[43]
- Professional codes of conduct usually allow for breaking of medical confidentiality in the case of considered assessments of dangerous driving when such drivers will not cease driving.
- Courts in the UK have considered that doctors are bound to advise patients on conditions that may impair safe driving.[44]

REFERENCES

1. *Active Ageing: a policy framework*. Geneva: World Health Organization; 2002.
2. *Report of the Second World Assembly on Ageing*. New York, NY: United Nations; 2002.
3. Russell C, O'Neill D. Developing an ethics of competence, care, and communication. *Ir Med J*. 2009; **102**(3): 69–70.
4. O'Neill D. More mad and more wise. *Accid Anal Prev*. 2012; **49**: 263–5.
5. Marmot M, Wilkinson RG. *Social Determinants of Health*. Oxford; New York: Oxford University Press; 1999.
6. Hjorthol R. Transport resources, mobility and unmet transport needs in old age. *Ageing and Society*. 2013; **33**: 1190–211.
7. Millar WJ. Older drivers: a complex public health issue. *Health Rep*. 1999; **11**(2): 59–71[English]; 67–82 [French].
8. *Ageing and Transport: mobility needs and safety issues*. Paris: Organisation for Economic Co-operation and Development; 2001.
9. Hakamies-Blomqvist L, Ukkonen T, O'Neill D. Driver ageing does not cause higher accident rates per mile. *Transport Res Part F, Traffic Psychol Behav*. 2002; **5**: 271–4.
10. Langford J, Methorst R, Hakamies-Blomqvist L. Older drivers do not have a high crash risk: a replication of low mileage bias. *Accid Anal Prev*. 2006; **38**(3): 574–8.

11. McGwin G Jr, Sims RV, Pulley L, *et al*. Relations among chronic medical conditions, medications, and automobile crashes in the elderly: a population-based case-control study. *Am J Epidemiol*. 2000; **152**(5): 424–31.

12. Redelmeier DA, Yarnell CJ, Tibshirani RJ. Physicians' warnings for unfit drivers and risk of road crashes. *N Engl J Med*. 2013; **368**(1): 87–8.

13. MacMahon M, O'Neill D, Kenny RA. Syncope: driving advice is frequently overlooked. *Postgrad Med J*. 1996; **72**(851): 561–3.

14. Frampton A. Who can drive home from the emergency department? A questionnaire based study of emergency physicians' knowledge of DVLA guidelines. *Emerg Med*. 2003; **20**(6): 526–30.

15. Akiyama T, Powell JL, Mitchell LB, *et al*. The antiarrhythmics versus implantable defibrillators I. Resumption of driving after life-threatening ventricular tachyarrhythmia. *N Engl J Med*. 2001; **345**(6): 391–7.

16. Bansch D, Brunn J, Castrucci M, *et al*. Syncope in patients with an implantable cardioverter-defibrillator: incidence, prediction and implications for driving restrictions. *J Am Coll Cardiol*. 1998; **31**(3): 608–15.

17. Owsley C, Stalvey B, Wells J, *et al*. Older drivers and cataract: driving habits and crash risk. *J Gerontol A Biol Sci Med Sci*. 1999; **54**(4): M203–11.

18. Monestam E, Wachmeister L. Impact of cataract surgery on the visual ability of the very old. *Am J Ophthalmol*. 2004; **137**(1): 145–55.

19. Wood JM, Carberry TP. Bilateral cataract surgery and driving performance. *Br J Ophthalmol*. 2006; **90**(10): 1277–80.

20. Cranney AB, Harrison A, Ruhland L, *et al*. Driving problems in patients with rheumatoid arthritis. *J Rheumatol*. 2005; **32**(12): 2337–42.

21. Thevenon A, Grimbert P, Dudenko P, *et al*. Polarthrite rhumatoïde et conduite automobile. *Rev Rhum Mal Osteoartic*. 1989; **56**: 101–3.

22. Jones JG, McCann J, Lassere MN. Driving and arthritis. *Br J Rheumatology*. 1991; **30**: 361–4.

23. McGwin G, Sims RV, Pulley L, *et al*. Diabetes and automobile crashes in the elderly: a population-based case-control study. *Diabetes Care*. 1999; **22**(2): 220–7.

24. Driver and Vehicle Licensing Agency. *At a Glance*. Swansea: DVLA; 2013.

25. Austroads. *Assessing Fitness to Drive*. Sydney: Austroads; 2012.

26. Canadian Medical Association. *CMA Drivers Guide: determining medical fitness to drive*. 8th ed. Ottawa: CMA; 2013.

27. Carr D, Schwartzberg JG, Manning L, *et al*. *Physician's Guide to Assessing and Counseling Older Drivers*. 2nd ed. Washington, DC: National Highway Traffic Safety Administration; 2010.

28. Breen DA, Breen DP, Moore JW, *et al*. Driving and dementia. *BMJ*. 2007; **334**(7608): 1365–9.

29. Howe E. Improving treatments for patients who are elderly and have dementia. *J Clin Ethics*. 2000; **11**: 291–303.

30. Maguire CP, Kirby M, Coen R, *et al*. Family members' attitudes toward telling the patient with Alzheimer's disease their diagnosis. *BMJ*. 1996; **313**(7056): 529–30.

31. Turnbull Q, Wolf AM, Holroyd S. Attitudes of elderly subjects toward "truth telling" for the diagnosis of Alzheimer's disease. *J Geriatr Psychiatry Neurol*. 2003; **16**(2): 90–3.

32. Bahro M, Silber E, Box P, *et al*. Giving up driving in Alzheimer's disease: an integrative therapeutic approach. *Int J Geriatric Psychiatry*. 1995; **10**: 871–4.

33. *At the Crossroads: a guide to Alzheimer's disease, dementia and driving*. Hartford, CT: Hartford Foundation; 2007.

34. Vernon DD, Diller EM, Cook LJ, *et al.* Evaluating the crash and citation rates of Utah drivers licensed with medical conditions, 1992–1996. *Accid Anal Prev.* 2002; **34**(2): 237–46.

35. Foley DJ, Heimovitz HK, Guralnik JM, *et al.* Driving life expectancy of persons aged 70 years and older in the United States. *Am J Public Health.* 2002; **92**(8): 1284–9.

36. Freund K, Vine J. Aging, Mobility, and the Model T: Approaches to Smart Community Transportation. *Generations.* 2010; **34**(3): 76–81.

37. Choi M, Adams KB, Kahana E. The impact of transportation support on driving cessation among community-dwelling older adults. *J Gerontol B Psychol Sci Soc Sci.* 2012; **67**(3): 392–400.

38. Johnson JE. Informal social support networks and the maintenance of voluntary driving cessation by older rural women. *J Community Health Nurs.* 2008; **25**(2): 65–72.

39. Janke MK. Assessing older drivers: two studies. *J Saf Res.* 2001; **32**(1): 43–74.

40. Simpson CS, Hoffmaster B, Mitchell LB, *et al.* Mandatory physician reporting of drivers with cardiac disease: ethical and practical considerations. *Can J Cardiol.* 2004; **20**(13): 1329–34.

41. Drazkowski JF, Neiman ES, Sirven JI, *et al.* Frequency of physician counseling and attitudes toward driving motor vehicles in people with epilepsy: comparing a mandatory-reporting with a voluntary-reporting state. *Epilepsy Behav.* 2010; **19**(1): 52–4.

42. Remillard GM, Zifkin BG, Andermann F. Epilepsy and motor vehicle driving: a symposium held in Quebec City, November 1998. *Can J Neurol Sci.* 2002; **29**(4): 315–25.

43. O'Neill J. *McGarvey [a minor] v Barr*. [2011] IEHC 461. Dublin; 2011.

44. Strawford G. Driving license revoked. *J MDU.* 1999; **15**: 18.

CHAPTER 12

Achieving a good death

Jim Eccles and Gurcharan S Rai

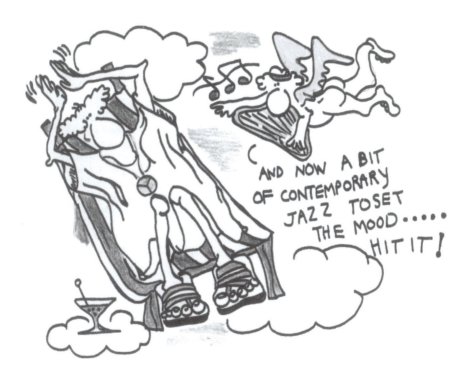

INTRODUCTION

There are between 50 000 and 100 000 'sudden' deaths in the UK each year due to natural causes, with the usual underlying pathologies being coronary artery disease, massive stroke and pulmonary embolism. Of the expected deaths many are foreseeable, with heart disease, cancer, stroke and respiratory disease being the major killers. A mercifully rapid final illness after enjoyment of an active life almost to the end is highly desirable, but in old age this is often not the outcome.

The time to die

The natural time to die is when the body can no longer sustain life, and this is usually in old age, since almost 80% of deaths in the UK occur in people over 65 years of age. Doctors who have the means to preserve organ function may need to ask themselves whether they are simply supporting vital physiological processes, or actually prolonging the process of dying.

The place to die

Most people, if asked, feel that they would prefer to die in their own homes, but the majority of us in the event die in institutions. Over half (54%) of all deaths occur in National Health Service (NHS) hospitals, 13% in private hospitals, residential care homes and nursing homes, and 4% in hospices. The remaining 29% occur in private households or elsewhere, such as in public places. To a varying extent, the doctor may have some influence over both where and how his or her patient dies. The Advance Care Planning guidance issued as part of the NHS End of Life Care Programme[1] emphasises the patient's right to choose where they wish to be cared for, at the end of life.

The way to die

There are many aspects of how we die, and here the doctor may have an important role. Three principles proposed by Jeffery and Millard[2] provide the doctor with tools to solve moral dilemmas at the end of life. These are as follows.

1. Treatment of patients must reflect the inherent dignity of every person irrespective of age, debility, dependence, race, colour or creed. The basis of the ancient Hippocratic oath is respect for the person as an individual in all aspects of medical and nursing management, including the period when withdrawal of treatment is being considered. The value of the person does not depend on whether treatment is useful or not.
2. Actions taken must reflect the needs of the patient where he or she is. Doctors' actions should not only display the highest standards of professional behaviour but also consider perceived burdens and benefits to the patient, the patient's family, professional health carers and the community.
3. Decisions taken must value the person and accept human mortality. Although it is the doctor's duty to do no harm, it is not his or her duty to preserve life at all costs. When a medical treatment or intervention is no longer appropriate to sustain life, or the means used to sustain life are out of proportion to the life achieved, death should be accepted and allowed to take its course.

If the patient can make meaningful choices about the nature of such treatment options, then the patient's own views should be sought, especially if those choices involve subjective judgements about the 'quality' of the life that remains.

DILEMMAS FACED BY DOCTORS WHEN DEALING WITH DEATH

Should the doctor tell or not tell?

This question relates to both diagnosis and prognosis. According to the General Medical Council (GMC),[3] doctors should share with the patient whatever the patient needs or wants to know, especially in the context of treatment decisions. The GMC advises doctors not to make assumptions about the information that an individual patient might want or need. We may simply tell the patient of our suspicion that there is something serious going on until that suspicion has been confirmed. Otherwise we could unnecessarily alarm the patient by sharing a wide differential diagnosis, which may unreasonably remove hope at an early stage. However, although patients have a right to know, perhaps they also have a right not to know. We are all familiar with patients who seem to desist pointedly from asking anything that could lead to a disclosure of the diagnosis. This plea not to be told should be respected, although opportunities to ask questions should continue to be offered. Sometimes it is a close relative who requests that the truth be withheld – 'She's always been terrified of cancer, doctor. She'd simply give up if she knew.' Such requests are usually misguided, and most patients can come to terms with the reality much better once it has been brought out into the open. Furthermore, a web of deceit puts family relationships under a great strain. When the patient is dying, it is particularly appropriate that the patient should set the pace of the discussions about prognosis. One of the most difficult aspects of these discussions is the degree of uncertainty involved, but if we can share at least what we know, we can help our patients to make timely choices about their own palliative care.

Who should tell?

Ideally, this person should be a trusted and familiar doctor or nurse in the presence of someone who is particularly close to the patient. All too often it turns out to be a stranger in the outpatient clinic or a hospital ward, and every effort should be made to avoid this.

Breaking bad news

Although they are not very strongly evidence based, here are a few guidelines for performing this unwelcome task in a kind and courteous way.

➤ Do not strive for too much detachment – patients and their relatives seem to appreciate it if the doctor or nurse is affected emotionally.

➤ Try not to kill all hope, or to give too precise a forecast of the duration of the illness. Offer a second opinion if one is wanted.

➤ Sit down to indicate that you have time for discussion. Do not be afraid of eye contact, appropriate physical contact or silence. Describe your findings, the possible actions and the reasons for the prognosis.

➤ Undertake to continue support and relieve symptoms. It is essential that the patient does not feel abandoned.

Consequent 'end-of-life decisions'

Patients may have conditions that severely limit both the duration and the quantity of expected life, such as a disseminated malignancy, a gangrenous leg or severe cardiac failure. They may have conditions that limit the experience and quality of life, such as end-stage dementia or recurrent and severe stroke disease. In such situations it becomes reasonable to emphasise the relief of distressing symptoms and the preservation of dignity.

THE PATIENT IN THE COMMUNITY

Should a medical emergency arise in the care of a dying patient, general practitioners (GPs) need to think long and hard before sending the patient into hospital. If they decide to do so, then they need to make it clear to the receiving doctor that the primary reason for admission is to access more intense nursing support, or specialist advice, rather than 'heroic' intervention. This is an important time to consider the locally available alternative models of palliative care at home, and some out-of-hours primary care services are now involved in making these choices more accessible. In the case of patients living in nursing homes, it is important that any advance care plans include the consideration of locally available options for continuing palliative care in the home, if the patient wants to avoid further hospital admission. The medical director and director of health protection, Public Health, England recommends influenza immunisation for older people, and although patients should be assessed for this in light of their individual prognosis, the impact on other vulnerable older people (such as fellow residents in a care home) of a failure to immunise should also be considered.

THE HOSPITAL PATIENT

Decisions about whether or not to subject patients to attempted cardiopulmonary resuscitation, or critical care support, should be taken in the context of their overall prognosis. In the case of patients receiving palliative care, it is particularly important to approach such decisions with sensitivity and tact. In hospital, the usual course is to record a resuscitation status in the notes. This is sensible, because in the event of a cardiac arrest there is no time to mull over the pros and cons of cardiopulmonary resuscitation. The most senior doctor available makes the decision[4] after discussion with the rest of the team, the patient if he or she is able to participate in decision-making, and the family in the case of a person who is incapacitated. It is not necessary to discuss futile interventions with a patient, but if it is thought that treatment decisions will depend on the anticipated result in terms of quality of life, then the patient should be consulted. The emphasis that is placed on recording the patient's resuscitation status should not prevent us from addressing those other treatment decisions that may be even more relevant to patients nearing the end of life, such as those concerned with nutritional support. A 'do not attempt resuscitation' (DNAR) decision does not imply that we are now only providing palliative rather than curative treatment; for instance, it should not automatically lead to the withholding of intravenous fluids or antibiotics. Particular attention should be paid to the sensitive decisions about whether or not to commence or continue the process of clinically assisted nutrition, and a second senior clinical opinion may be required in those circumstances. The guidance on end-of-life care issued by the GMC in 2010 emphasises the significance of good communication with patients and their families, even when such decisions are made on the grounds of clinical futility.[5]

PALLIATIVE CARE PATHWAYS

End-of-life care pathways were introduced to improve the quality of palliative care of dying patients, and to emulate the standard of care achieved in hospices. The most widely used pathway has been the Liverpool Care Pathway (LCP). In response to recent public concern about the use of the LCP in hospitals, the UK government established an independent review of the LCP. In particular, the review panel was asked to look at the quality of care of patients on the pathway, and the involvement of patients and their families in the process of making clinical decisions. The review report, published in July 2013, recommended that the LCP should be phased out and replaced with individual end-of-life care plans.[6]

ADVANCE CARE PLANNING

Some elderly people wish to declare in advance that, in the event of serious illness and incompetence to participate in decision-making because of unconsciousness or confusion, they would not wish for particular life-supporting measures. These advance decisions to refuse treatment should ideally be drawn up in consultation with their GP, and other health professionals involved in their care. The Mental Capacity Act 2005 put advance decisions on a statutory footing. However, under the Act an advance decision will not apply to life-sustaining treatment unless it includes a statement that it should apply 'even if life is at risk' and the statement is signed and witnessed.

Advance decisions present obvious practical difficulties. As a simple example, who will be aware of the decision if a person is rushed to hospital at night as an emergency? More fundamentally, it is impossible to envisage in advance every possible medical scenario that might arise. For these reasons, some people may choose to appoint an attorney to act on his or her behalf under a lasting power of attorney, but the attorney will only be able to make a healthcare decision once an individual becomes incapacitated (*see also* Chapter 9, 'Advance decisions/advance decisions to refuse treatment'). The National Council for Palliative Care has produced guidance for health and social care professionals,[7] so that they will be able to assist patients to complete an advance decision, and it includes a model advance decision form.

In the future, patients with a life-limiting illness may be given the opportunity to complete an electronically stored advance care plan, in consultation with the clinicians who are caring for them. If each plan was shared with other healthcare agencies, such as the ambulance service, then a decision about the patient's preferred place of care, for example, would be more transparent, and this could prevent an inappropriate journey to hospital at the end of a terminal illness. The Coordinate My Care initiative in London offers a new model of such a service that may soon be available throughout the NHS.[8]

THE ROLE OF CLOSE FRIENDS AND RELATIVES

It is obviously right for doctors to make themselves available to patients' families, and many complaints arise from poor communication between health service staff and patients' relatives. In the case of infants, the parents have a decision-making capacity, within reasonable limits. In the case of adults, the immediate family does not have a decision-making capacity, but the sensible doctor will listen attentively to their views. However, the ultimate responsibility for the decision is the doctor's. The motives of the relatives are in any case sometimes rather mixed. Those who demand that all possible life-saving measures should be taken may feel guilty after years of worry about whether they have neglected an ailing relative. Those who suggest that it would be kinder to withdraw further aggressive treatment may be desperate to get their hands on the inheritance!

The Mental Capacity Act 2005 provides guidance on decision-making on behalf of incompetent adults who require 'serious medical treatment'.

1. Consider if the decision can be delayed until the patient is capable of making the decision him- or herself. If not, move to the following step.
2. Enquire if the patient has a valid and applicable advance decision.
3. Enquire if the patient has appointed a lasting power of attorney for healthcare decisions.
4. If there is no one appropriate to act as a 'natural advocate' for the patient, request the appointment of an independent mental capacity advocate.
5. Where there is remaining disagreement about the patient's best interests, the decision should be referred to the Court of Protection.

EUTHANASIA

Traditionally, the term 'euthanasia', derived from the Greek words *eu* and *thanatos*, has simply meant 'a good death', but today it refers to the ending of life of a person who is suffering from advanced incurable illness, for his or her benefit, by another. What constitutes a 'good death'? The answer is three factors: the time to die, the place and the manner of death.

Definitions

➤ *Voluntary euthanasia*: the deliberate and intentional hastening of death at the request of the patient, who is seriously ill.

➤ *Involuntary euthanasia*: the ending of a person's life without seeking his or her opinion.

➤ *Non-voluntary euthanasia*: the ending of a person's life, for his or her own benefit, when that person cannot possess or express views about whether he or she lives or dies.

➤ *Physician-assisted suicide*: the patient takes by him- or herself deliberately lethal medication that has been prescribed or provided by the physician.

Euthanasia in the context of end-of-life care

The main decision confronting the doctor of a patient near the end of life is whether the aim should be palliation of symptoms or cure of the underlying cause. Most doctors subscribe to the traditional doctrine that good palliative care may involve gradually increasing the dosage of sedatives and analgesics with the aim of relieving suffering and distress, although this may have the unintended consequence of hastening the patient's death through depression of respiration, cough and movement (the so-called 'double effect'). In such cases, it is the doctor's intent that is crucial. It is important to understand that increasing the dosage of pain-killing drugs, such as morphine, does not necessarily hasten death. Sometimes it is found that controlling the pain reduces the need for sedation and enhances the duration and quality of life.

If a patient has a colonic carcinoma with widespread metastases that is now threatening to cause obstruction, a surgeon might perform a palliative bypass procedure, but no one would expect him or her to carry out a radical resection, on the grounds that it would be futile. In this situation, no one would use the term 'passive euthanasia'. If a patient with Down's syndrome were denied antibiotics for pneumonia, people might use that expression, although the most pressing question in such a case might be why a potentially life-prolonging treatment was withheld, and whether there was an element of discrimination. The term 'passive euthanasia' implies that decisions to withhold or withdraw life-prolonging treatment have been taken with the intention that the patient will die. Such decisions are specifically defined as being against the law in the UK in the case of incapacitated patients, according to the Mental Capacity Act 2005. Although some philosophers regard such withdrawals of treatment as 'passive euthanasia', the primary intention of the doctor is critical. If the doctor's intention is palliation and the medical intention of palliative care is the relief of distress, then treatment decisions may be based on a judgement of the value or futility of available treatment options, in the context of the patient's condition. An accurate assessment of the patient's mental and physical condition is therefore necessary, but there should be no attempt to judge the worth or futility of the patient's life, which is a matter for deeply personal and subjective consideration by the patient alone. The key question that doctors are expected to ask themselves in each case is therefore 'Is the treatment

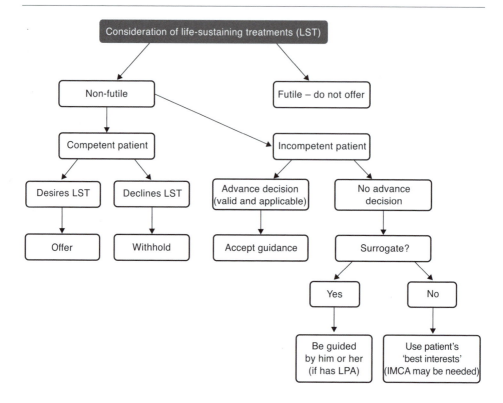

FIGURE 12.1 Consideration of life-sustaining treatment (LST) (IMCA = independent mental capacity advocate; LPA = lasting power of attorney)

worthwhile or futile?' and not 'Is the patient's life worthwhile or futile?' If the decision depends on the perceived quality of a patient's life after treatment, then every effort should be made to understand that life as viewed from the patient's own, unique perspective (*see* Figure 12.1).

Stopping treatment because a patient is dying, and stopping treatment because the doctor wants the patient to die are not the same thing. It is therefore important that doctors record not only their palliative care treatment plans but also the intention of those plans, in order to avoid misinterpretation of their motives. The practice of active euthanasia, on the other hand, implies an intention to hasten the death of the patient on the basis of the presumed benefit of hastening death. The Human Rights Act 1998 has been used on both sides of the debate surrounding euthanasia. It declares a right to life, but also states that people should not be subjected to inhuman or degrading treatment. The courts in the UK have not interpreted this as permitting the right of competent individuals to die by assisted suicide, and it is clear that both assisted suicide and euthanasia are still strictly against the law in the UK.

In 2010 the Director of Public Prosecutions published a policy on cases of assisted suicide, to clarify the circumstances in which a prosecution would be pursued. The factors in favour of a prosecution include circumstances in which the suspect had pressured the victim to commit suicide or had stood to gain in some way from the death of the victim. There is also a specific reference to suspects who may have assisted the victim in their capacity as doctors or nurses, and that is regarded as being a factor in favour of prosecution.[9] The GMC has also published specific guidance to doctors on how to deal with a patient who seeks advice about assistance to die, while ensuring that their response does not contravene the law by encouraging or assisting the patient to commit suicide.[10]

One argument against euthanasia is that of the 'slippery slope' – for example, that there might be a gradual moral decline of society through unethical actions that become increasingly acceptable (*see* Box 12.1).

BOX 12.1 The 'slippery slope' in end-of-life care

Civilised society (respect for life)

Assisted suicide (competent patient seeks help to commit suicide)

Voluntary euthanasia (competent patient expresses wish to be put to death)

Altruistic euthanasia (request for euthanasia for the benefit of others)

Dutiful euthanasia (based on the social acceptance of a 'duty to die')

Non-voluntary euthanasia (incompetent patient unable to express opinions)

Involuntary euthanasia (social decision, patient's opinion not sought)

Barbaric society (no respect for life)

RELIGION

Although our society has become increasingly secular, for many people a good death will involve respect for their religious beliefs. Religion can offer some understanding of mortality, and the ceremonies and rituals that surround dying can be a comfort both to patients and to their families. An understanding of religious beliefs is useful for comprehending attitudes to death, and an appreciation of the different customs is important for those involved in the care of dying patients. The history of the hospice movement demonstrates the close involvement of religious organisations in the voluntary provision of palliative care in the community, and this tradition continues to this day.

Most religions promote the protection and care of those who are dying and therefore forbid euthanasia. The monotheistic faiths, such as Christianity, Judaism and Islam, teach that life is sacred, as it is given by God (the Creator), and therefore intentionally ending life is prohibited. While these religions teach that all life has a value, they also acknowledge that life need not be preserved at all costs. There is recognition of the compassionate necessity to alleviate suffering and preserve dignity. As always, there is a spectrum of beliefs within these faiths. For example, the Orthodox Jewish tradition attaches much more importance to prolonging life than do other faiths. In Buddhism and Hinduism, there is a little more ambiguity because of the belief in reincarnation. Hastening the end of life would interfere with this process and would go against the principle of *ahimsa* (doing no harm). However, there is a distinction between selfish reasons for ending life and spiritual or compassionate reasons, such as the relieving of distress for relatives. These are great simplifications, but in general there is a consensus of religious opinion against euthanasia.

CASE HISTORIES

A number of case histories are given here that illustrate some of the situations that may arise as death approaches. The patients are all elderly, representing the age group in which the large majority of deaths occur in the developed world. The real message behind these cases is that end-of-life decisions are often difficult, and there may be no clear-cut right or wrong answers. The patient's autonomy is paramount and the patient's views should always be respected, when the necessary mental capacity has been demonstrated. Even when mental capacity appears to be impaired, we should listen hard to our patients, in order to understand those preferences that can still be expressed.

CASE 12.1

Mr A, aged 82 years, was admitted with right lower lobe pneumonia. Two years previously he had a stroke and was profoundly dysarthric and unable to swallow solids or fluids without aspirating or choking. Two weeks ago his wife had died, but he had an elderly dog of which he was inordinately fond. His presumed aspiration pneumonia responded well to antibiotics, but he pulled out a nasogastric tube and refused a percutaneous endoscopic gastrostomy (PEG). He wrote several pathetic notes to the medical staff begging to be allowed home. It was felt that he was not truly depressed, but that death by dehydration and starvation alone in his cold and cheerless home would be a very sad fate. After discussion with his GP, and a careful assessment of his mental capacity, his request was acceded to, and he was doing well several months later.

Comments
- Competent patients are entitled to make 'unwise' decisions.
- Patients may survive decisions to 'eat and drink at risk'.
- The elderly thrive far better in their own homes.
- Best interests are personal. (Two patients with identical medical conditions may have entirely different best interests.)

CASE 12.2

Mrs B, aged 80 years, was admitted via the accident and emergency department from her residential care home where she had sustained a number of falls. Two years previously she had been diagnosed as having severe dementia, and she was now agitated and aggressive, incontinent, and variably mobile with a frame and some assistance. On his ward round, the geriatrician recorded a DNAR order in her notes. The care staff from her home reviewed her, but felt unable to have her back, so attempts were made to find a nursing home placement. One morning Mrs B choked and aspirated, and the house officer initiated intravenous antibiotics, despite which she died. Her son subsequently complained on the grounds that:
- the DNAR decision was unjustified
- it should have been discussed with him
- it may have been made simply because the hospital needed the bed (!).

Comment
- A DNAR decision does not necessarily involve other non-treatment decisions unless specified.
- Even if a DNAR decision is made on the grounds of medical futility, it is good practice to keep the family closely informed if the patient has lost the mental capacity to participate in discussion.

CASE 12.3

Mrs C, aged 78 years, who was residing in a nursing home because of multiple strokes, was sent into hospital by a visiting GP because she had ceased to eat or drink. She was profoundly dehydrated, severely dysphagic, had an indwelling catheter, and the electrolytes showed a sodium level of 183 mmol/L with a urea level of 48.9 mmol/L. She received intravenous rehydration, as the on-call team felt that this was the GP's intention and the consultant doing the 'post-take ward round' decided to send her back to the familiar surroundings of the nursing home. However, during an acrimonious interview her six sons and daughters insisted that their mother was mentally intact, valued her life, and would wish for PEG feeding, a request to which the consultant reluctantly acceded.

Comment
- You are treating the patient, not the family, but you should gracefully accept that they often know the patient better than you do.
- The sight of a loved one in a physically vulnerable state may trigger an understandable but highly protective response.
- Nutritional support in dysphagic stroke survivors is the most sensitive issue in the management of stroke patients. Current guidance is to feed with a nasogastric tube, and later convert to PEG feeding if dysphagia persists (in

order to maintain nutrition rather than to guarantee protection of the airway), except in cases where the prognostic indicators are so bad that prolongation of life is contrary to the patient's best interests.

- Try to encourage the family to consider the issue in context of the overall prognosis.
- If discussion with the family becomes difficult, an early offer of a second opinion may reassure them that we are considering all aspects of the case.
- If the patient recovers, try to establish an agreed care plan that incorporates a strategy for managing similar crises in the future.

CASE 12.4

Mr D, aged 78 years, was sent into hospital with rapidly increasing breathless-ness. He was found to be cachectic and to have a large pleural effusion with a 'white-out' on the X-ray. The fluid was bloodstained, but no malignant cells were found, so the respiratory physician was contacted. He suggested further aspiration for cytology and, if the result was still negative, a pleural biopsy after stopping the warfarin that Mr D was still taking for previous pulmonary emboli. This procedure was performed a week later, by which time Mr D had become progressively weaker, and he died shortly thereafter.

Comment

- The consideration of what investigations may be in the patient's best interests depends on doctors having clear goals in terms of possible benefits, and a clear understanding of the risks involved.
- These should be shared with the patient (if mentally competent) or those people who are close to the patient.
- Our discussions need to include an honest expression of any diagnostic or therapeutic uncertainty.

SUMMARY OF END-OF-LIFE DECISIONS

➤ Will further investigation clarify the overall management?
➤ Information should be shared with the patient and/or the family.
➤ Resuscitation decisions should be taken in context of the overall prognosis.
➤ Is the aim of treatment a cure of underlying pathology, or primarily palliative?
➤ Both UK law and the latest medical professional guidance in the UK support a distinction between the withdrawal of active treatment as part of palliative care and the intentional ending of human life.

REFERENCES

1. *NHS Choices. End of Life Care: planning ahead for the end of life. London: NHS Choices; n.d.* Available at: www.nhs.uk/Planners/end-of-life-care/Pages/planning-ahead.aspx (accessed 6 November 2013).
2. Jeffery P, Millard PH. An ethical framework for clinical decision-making at the end of life. *J R Soc Med.* 1997; **90**(9): 504–6.
3. General Medical Council. *Consent Guidance: patients and doctors making decisions together.* Manchester: GMC; 2008. Available at: www.gmc-uk.org/guidance/ethical_guidance/consent_guidance/contents.asp (accessed 6 November 2013).
4. British Medical Association; Resuscitation Council (UK); Royal College of Nursing. *Decisions Relating to Cardiopulmonary Resuscitation.* London: BMA; 2007. Available at: www.resus.org.uk/pages/dnar.htm (accessed 26 March 2014).
5. General Medical Council. *Treatment and Care Towards the End of Life: good practice in decision making.* Manchester: GMC; 2010. Available at: www.gmc-uk.org/guidance/ethical_guidance/end_of_life_care.asp (accessed 26 March 2014).
6. Department of Health. *Review of Liverpool Care Pathway for Dying Patients.* London: DH; 2013. Available at: www.gov.uk/government/publications/review-of-liverpool-care-pathway-for-dying-patients (accessed 6 November 2013).
7. National Council for Palliative Care. *Advance Decisions to Refuse Treatment: a guide for health and social care professionals.* London: NCPC; 2008. Available at: www.ncpc.org.uk/publication/advance-decisions-refuse-treatment-guide-health-and-social-care-professionals (accessed 26 March 2014).
8. http://coordinatemycare.co.uk
9. Crown Prosecution Service. *Policy for Prosecutors in Respect of Cases of Encouraging or Assisting Suicide.* London: Crown Prosecution Service; 2010.
10. General Medical Council. *When a Patient Seeks Advice or Information about Assistance to Die.* London: GMC; 2013.

CHAPTER 13

Religious beliefs of patients and end-of-life decisions

Aza Abdulla and Gurcharan S Rai

INTRODUCTION

It is important for doctors to have knowledge and appreciation of differences encountered in religious and social attitudes to deliver a compassionate care. Decision-making, particularly in relation to resuscitation and care at end of life, requires the doctor to have knowledge of his or her patients' beliefs. This chapter will discuss the views and beliefs of common religions that may affect clinical decision-making, particularly at the end of life.

THE NEED FOR SPIRITUAL AND RELIGIOUS CARE

Studies have reported that between 33% and 77% of patients are interested in having clinicians attend to their spiritual needs.[1] The physician's duty of beneficence requires respect for patient spirituality and many organisations have recommended attention to the spiritual and religious needs of patients as an ethical obligation and an essential aspect of clinical practice.[2,3] Therefore, it is important that doctors and other healthcare professionals are able to discuss spiritual and religious issues with their patients.

RELIGION VERSUS SPIRITUALITY

In academic circles, it has become increasingly common to accept spirituality and religion as distinct but overlapping entities. Religion can be understood as a set of beliefs and practices shared by a community, whereas spirituality is commonly defined as a person's existential relationship with God or the Transcendent. Spirituality relates to the way in which people understand and live their lives in relation to their core beliefs and values and their perception of ultimate meaning. Spirituality is not confined to religion; it may be attained through interaction with nature, the arts or a humanist approach, especially in non-believers. Despite this, however, in reality this distinction – especially in the older religious person – is quite blurred and the two terms are in fact used interchangeably.[4]

ASSESSMENT AND MANAGEMENT OF SPIRITUAL AND RELIGIOUS ISSUES

A survey of medical residents conducted by the American Board of Internal Medicine found that 85% of residents feel uncomfortable talking to patients about their wishes and moral values and about dying. The reluctance to talk about spiritual issues with patients is due to several reasons. Foremost of these has been the lack of training during undergraduate and postgraduate training. Until recently, medical training has focused on healing illness and physical management, with the result that doctors have come to believe that it is not their role to get involved in spiritual and evangelical discussions with patients. This traditional training has resulted in a lack of confidence, such that doctors may feel overwhelmed and unsure how to respond if patients raise spiritual matters.

Clinicians should be able to elicit a spiritual history from the patient. Even if a patient's religion dictates a certain belief or practice, it does not necessarily mean that the patient will hold that belief, and very few patients are offended by gentle non-judgemental questioning on their religious and spiritual beliefs. Several assessment tools have been developed, although the narrative approach is probably the most likely way to consolidate good rapport with the patient and, in certain instances, his or her family. Simple open-ended questions may provide a less formal approach to obtain the necessary information. Examples of such questions include the following: Are you a religious person? Do you have any spiritual or religious requirements that the hospital can arrange for you? Are there any spiritual beliefs that you wish to discuss? Would you like to see a chaplain or someone from pastoral care?

The information could be acquired during the initial history taking, in the context of breaking bad news or during a medical crisis – for example, deterioration in clinical condition. Respect for the patient requires attention to detail and careful listening, and the choice of words is important when talking to the patient or to his or her family.

The role of the clinician is to clarify the patient's concerns, beliefs and spiritual needs, and to attempt to establish trust where patient and family can share their deepest concerns and not feel embarrassed to ask for help.

The importance of a multidisciplinary approach to spiritual needs cannot be overstated, especially in cases of spiritual distress, when appropriate referral should be made to spiritual care providers (e.g. chaplain, other clergy), who can address these issues in depth.

END-OF-LIFE (INCLUDING RESUSCITATION) VIEWS OF THE COMMON RELIGIONS

Religion for many people provides a meaning for one's existence, which often becomes more important around the end of life. The physician should be aware of the basic differences between religions in their approach to end-of-life issues.

Buddhism

Buddhism is a moderate religion, but unlike most of the other religions, there is no central authority to pronounce on doctrine and ethics. In practice, local customs will often be more important in the relationship between physician and patient than Buddhist doctrine. Therefore, attitudes towards end of life may be different among Tibetan, Indian, Thai and Western Buddhists. Hence, it is extremely important to enquire about the specific attitudes held by the patient and family, even though most Buddhist communities share certain attitudes.

Buddhism emphasises compassion and respect for life. There is general understanding that both assisted suicide and euthanasia are immoral and prohibited even on grounds of compassion. However, Buddhists do not believe in prolonging life at all costs. Death is inevitable and attempts to preserve life when no recovery is in sight deny human mortality. In such a situation it is justifiable to withdraw, or for the patient to refuse, treatment if it is futile.

Buddhism believes in reincarnation. At the time of death the body and mind go through a state of dissolution that continues for up to 3 days after breathing stops. At that point the mind, now in a subtle state, separates from the body, taking with it all the imprints from the life that it embodied and which it adds to the previous ones. Following a period lasting up to 7 weeks, a place of rebirth is found, which is determined by the state of karma, and a new material life begins.

Crucial in this whole process is the state of mind at the time of death, because it determines the new reborn state. If the mind is in a state of anger and fear, this will predispose to an unhappy or lower state of rebirth. Therefore, it is important to help the person die with spiritual thoughts and a peaceful, unclouded and clear mind. Some Buddhists may be unwilling to accept sedatives or pain relief that may impair their mental or sensory capacities.

The recital of prayers, spiritual music, burning of incense and the presence of family members or friends is important for the religious patient around the time of death, to aid in making the transition from this life to the next as meaningful as possible. It is helpful for nurses and doctors looking after the patient to recognise the spiritual importance of this transition.

Christianity

Christianity is probably the most diverse religion, as it encompasses a cluster of religious groups, each with its own dominion and theology, all under the one umbrella of Christianity. Anglican, Roman Catholic, Eastern Orthodox,

Protestant, Lutheran, Unitarian, Mormon, and Baptist are examples of the main denominations. Physicians should recognise that Christianity is no single order and that each group will have its own directives, beliefs and practices. The manner in which members of one denomination regard the practice of others varies from acceptance to denial and refusal.

Furthermore, Christianity in its broad sense has become so much part of Western society (both law and culture) that separating its secularised influence from the actual spiritual teaching is difficult.[10]

Christianity sees death as a fact of life (Hebrews 9:27) and that there is 'a time to be born, and a time to die' (Ecclesiastes 3:2). Christianity believes in divine forgiveness and that salvation will be available through death and prayer. After death we shall be called to account and will be judged by our past deeds. Death is therefore seen as a period for moral reckoning and so may be a cause of anxiety and fear.

There is considerable respect for human life in Christianity, as people are created in the image of God (Jesus Christ as the incarnation of God). Life is a gift from God and individuals are accountable to God for the life given to them. As a general rule, Christianity prohibits actions that intentionally cause death. Although people are seen as stewards rather than owners of their bodies, it is not an absolute good to be preserved at any cost; dignity of the human person lies above all.

Pain and suffering is not without meaning in Catholic bioethics. It construes a redemptive nature, but this belief does not imply that pain relief should be withheld.

If treatment only postpones the moment of death, then it may be appropriate for a competent patient with decision-making capacity to refuse medical intervention. If the patient is incapable of making these decisions, family members or advocates may step in to make these decisions in the best interests of the patient.

Christians regard last rites as an integral part of their relationship with God. Quite often it is the priest from the patient's own denomination who should perform the last rites. The presence of a chaplain or priest should be offered around the time of death. At this time the sacraments become of particular importance to strengthen the patient's faith. This includes formal confession, receiving communion and final anointing. In Catholicism, the Sacrament of the Anointing of the Sick is a sign of God's presence in the life of the seriously ill and dying person. The sacrament is a source of grace and strength. Another ritual is the viaticum, a series of prayers and a blessing for the passage to death and eternal life, along with the reception of Holy Communion. The concern for final repentance may, at least in theory, affect the amount of sedation needed to control pain. However, the use of analgesia and sedation to avoid or reduce pain is permissible, if it does not take away the final opportunity of repentance by reducing consciousness.

Withdrawal of artificial feeding and hydration at end of life is an issue of debate with much controversy. Similarly, the view on physician-assisted suicide and euthanasia is also diverse, as opinions vary even within the same denomination. Some are clearly opposed while others may see it as a patient's choice.

Because beliefs and attitudes vary among the different denominations, it is important to develop an understanding of the particular patient's Christian values through enquiring and listening.

Hinduism

The concept of karma, reincarnation, and absorption into ultimate reality and enlightenment exists in both Hinduism and Buddhism. Karma refers to one's acts and thoughts, and it has consequences on the next life; it decides a good or bad rebirth. Pain and suffering may be explained by past karma. However, suffering is seen as purifying, and a dying patient in pain may refuse treatment in order to die with a clear mind – pain expurgating sin. Suicide is morally wrong because of the karmic effect on the next life. Euthanasia is also prohibited, and those involved 'will take on the remaining karma of the patient'.[11]

The concept of good death and bad death in Hinduism deserves attention. A good death is timely and in the right place, usually in the patient's own surrounding. In contrast, a bad death is violent and unprepared, at the wrong time, or associated with body functions such as vomiting and incontinence. This probably implies suffering. A good death requires the right rituals to see the soul on its way. Failure to do so can result in a bad death; the soul fails to move on, haunting the family and risking bad luck for generations to come.

In both Hinduism and Sikhism, a 'do not attempt resuscitation' order is usually accepted or desired because death should be peaceful, and artificially or mechanically sustained life is of little value.[12]

The ritual of chanting prayers, reciting, to ensure the dying patient focuses on God (Ishvara) are usually only carried out when death is imminent. Moving the patient to lie on the ground, with the head to the north and wetting the lips with holy Ganges water and a basil leaf placed in the mouth just before death is expected. The act of penance may be led by a priest or conducted by the family and continues until after death when they bid farewell to the deceased. Not allowing these rituals may leave a long-lasting effect on the family of the dying person.

The family have a duty to assist the dying person but they also have a duty to protect him or her from bad news. Therefore, a tension may evolve between autonomy for the patient and knowledge of outcome to prepare for a good end and the protection that the family like to offer to prevent the patient from giving up hope and thereby accepting a premature death.

Islam

Islamic teaching according to the Qur'an dictates that 'He (Allah) who brought disease also sent cure'; therefore, patients and health providers should seek treatment and prevent premature death. There is an obligation to save and prolong life.

On the other hand, Islam acknowledges that death is inevitable, everyone will face death and that 'a person dies when it is written' (Qur'an 29:57). It dictates that the life of a human being is sacred and no other human being has the right to end it (except as penalty for murder). On these grounds, assisted suicide and euthanasia in Islam is prohibited, although an exception is in cases of severe intractable pain where the physician, to relieve distress, can prescribe and administer pain relief that might carry the risk of shortening life. However the Qur'an maintains that pain is inflicted to attest faith and therefore in some patients it may be endured with perseverance, declining pain relief treatment.

Muslim jurists have ruled that life support once started cannot be switched off, unless it is certain beyond doubt that death is inevitable. Muslim jurists have also declared in a fatwa (religious decree) that three knowledgeable and trustworthy physicians need to agree that the patient's condition is hopeless, before life-supporting treatment including ventilation can be withheld or withdrawn. The family will be informed but they will not be involved in the decision. If the family disagree, then the care of patient can be transferred to another specialist.

It has been reported that this approach in Saudi Arabia has resulted in a dramatic reduction in futile cardiopulmonary resuscitation.[7] In Islamic teaching, the interest of the group or community takes precedence over the interest of the individual.[8] This has raised issues about the use of expensive treatment for individuals with uncertain outcome depriving the public of better use of resources, especially at times of economic difficulties.[7]

There still remains a certain degree of paternalism and the authoritative role of the doctor in Islamic countries, but is by no means universal practice. In Western countries, Muslim scholars maintain that a collective decision not to prolong life (and to withdraw futile treatment) in cases of terminal illness, through consultation with all those providing care and the family, is important.[9]

The patient may decline treatment if its purpose is to delay death. It is also the right of a competent patient to make his or her own decision regarding a 'do not attempt resuscitation' order. However, in Islamic ethics a person's welfare is closely linked with his or her family. Therefore, the principle of autonomy is not invoked when consultation with family members is undertaken to determine the course of action in matters of end-of-life decisions.

When death becomes inevitable, the patient should be allowed to die without unnecessary procedures. While all ongoing medical treatments can be continued, no further or new attempts should be made to sustain artificial life support.[8]

At the time of death, orthodox Muslim tradition dictates that the body should be turned towards Mecca. If that is not possible, then the head is turned in that direction. Family members recite verses from the Qur'an.

Judaism

Halacha, the Jewish religious laws, provides guidance for most aspects of day-to-day life. In principle the human body belongs to God (Yahweh) and any act to desecrate the body is not allowed. Therefore, suicide, assisted suicide and euthanasia is prohibited. Similarly, the Orthodox view holds that any act to hasten death, including withdrawal of care that has already been instituted, is not allowed.

Treatment to provide comfort is permitted. This includes prescribing opiates that may risk hastening the patient's death, as long as the intention is not to kill but rather to alleviate pain.

The patient may decline life-prolonging treatment if it is futile, and it would indeed be proper not to treat if such treatment only prolongs the dying process. However, this is a decision that the patient or, if the patient is incompetent, his or her family should make.

Similar to Islamic faith, in Jewish sources, the doctor has much more authority to determine the appropriate course of treatment. The patient does have the right to choose the treatment, but he or she does not have the right to demand treatment that, in the judgement of the clinician, is medically futile or unwise. Patient autonomy in Orthodox practice is therefore more restricted, although this approach is more likely to be blurred, depending on the region and country, social background and family constructs. Current practice, especially in Western countries, entails a patient–doctor partnership.

The sanctity of life is a fundamental consideration and a basic part of the Jewish ethics. Here feeding and nutrition is considered a basic human requirement and should be pursued in a way similar to the management of pressure sores and general hygiene, both of which are continued until death. Therefore, feeding and nutrition should be considered (including nasogastric and gastrostomy feeding) unless the risks of such treatment outweigh the expected clinical benefits. This argument in the Orthodox Jewish doctrine extends to patients with terminal illness and even dementia.[5] A less restrictive opinion considers artificial feeding and hydration as medicine and therefore it may be withdrawn if recovery is unlikely.[6] However, at times these measures may come into conflict with patient autonomy. Therefore, in situations where death is certain, the wish of a competent patient to refuse treatment, including feeding, is respected on the grounds that it may prolong suffering without improving prognosis.

The doctrine commandment of 'do not stand idly by while your neighbour's blood is being spilled' does imply the need to intervene when a patient is seriously ill. This may be seen as a need to resuscitate all ill patients. However, Judaism recognises the inevitability of death. Furthermore, the code of Jewish law prohibits touching the body of a patient who is terminally ill and expected to die within a short period (usually 3 days), referred to as *goses*, for fear that movement may accelerate the time of death. Resuscitation in such situations is considered an intrusion on the dying person. Only when there is a reasonable expectation of improving outcome is resuscitation indicated.

Sikhism

Compared with the other religions outlined in this chapter, Sikhism is relatively new, dating to around 500 years ago. Sikhs believe in karma and reincarnation, in that the soul may be reborn many times as a human or an animal. Therefore, for Sikhs, death is not the end. The Sikh sacred text, the Guru Granth Sahib, declares that the body is just clothing for the soul and is discarded at death. The physical body is therefore perishable, but the soul is eternal. The soul is a part of God (the Creator) and yearns reunion with the Supreme Being. Liberation from the cycle of birth and death, from millions of life forms, is the basis of the Sikh understanding of the purpose of life. Human life is seen as the gift of the Divine, and its termination, a return to the Divine source.

The timing of birth and death should be left in the Creator's hands. Therefore, Sikhs are discouraged in their faith to terminate their lives before the will of God (the Creator) dictates. Similarly, assisted suicide and euthanasia are not encouraged.

Everything that happens is the will of God (the Creator). However, healing through prayer and medicine are both possible.

Baptised Sikhs, also known as members of the 'Khalsa', at all times wear on their person five religious symbols that are articles of faith. These articles of faith are known as the five Ks because their names all start with the letter 'k'. The five Ks are (1) uncut hair (kesh), a gift from God representing spirituality; (2) a wooden comb (kangha), which symbolises cleanliness; (3) a steel bracelet (kara), which represents self-restraint and link to God; (4) a short sword (kirpan), an emblem of courage and commitment to truth and justice; (5) a type of underwear (kachha or kacchera), which represents purity of moral character.

Sikhs view the individual in the context of his or her family. Thus, the person is seen not as autonomous but rather as intimately integrated with his or her extended family, caste and environment. This necessitates a holistic approach to ethical matters such as informed consent, one that includes the patient's societal context.

Around the time of death the patient or relatives may request the service of a Sikh priest. Hymns from the Guru Granth Sahib are recited and prayers are performed as an essential part of the patient's final days. The body of the deceased should be covered with clean linen and shrouded. If the deceased is wearing any of the five Ks, the articles should be kept intact and remain on the body.

CONCLUSION

It is impossible to cover every religion in a short chapter. Even within each religion there is a wide spectrum of followers, from the orthodox to the more liberal. The issues around end-of-life care for patients are intertwined. In addition to religion and faith, the advances in medical technology, the availability of evolving and effective treatment with the potential ability to prolong life, and social factors such as the cosmopolitan attitude of many immigrants as they settle in another geographical area, education and cultural background will all have an impact on end-of-life beliefs and attitudes.

Respect for patients mandates deference and attention to their specific religious needs, and this becomes especially important with end-of-life issues. Therefore, it is important to explore the patient's and the family's particular faith and religious position. An understanding of the patient's religion and spirituality will illuminate the clinician's views and improve patient–clinician interaction.

KEY POINTS

Buddhism

- Buddhism emphasises compassion and respect for life, although Buddhists do not believe in prolonging life at all costs. Death is inevitable and attempts to preserve life when no recovery is in sight deny human mortality. In such a situation it is justifiable to withdraw, or for the patient to refuse, treatment if it is futile.

Christianity

- Christianity sees death as a fact of life: there is 'a time to be born, and a time to die'. If treatment only postpones the moment of death, then it may be appropriate for a competent patient with decision-making capacity to refuse medical intervention.
- Because beliefs and attitudes vary among the different denominations, it is important to develop an understanding of the particular patient's Christian values through enquiring and listening.

Hinduism

- Hinduism includes the concept of good death and bad death. A good death is timely and in the right place, usually in the patient's own surrounding; in contrast, a bad death is violent and unprepared, at the wrong time, or associated with body functions such as vomiting and incontinence.

Islam

- While Islam dictates that human life is sacred and there is an obligation to save and prolong life, Islam also acknowledges that death is inevitable.
- When death becomes inevitable, the patient should be allowed to die without unnecessary procedures.

Judaism

- Under Halacha, the Jewish religious laws, the human body belongs to God (Yahweh) and any act to desecrate the body is not allowed. The Orthodox view holds that any act to hasten death, including withdrawal of care that has already been instituted, is not allowed. Treatment to provide comfort is permitted, as long as the intention is not to kill but rather to alleviate pain.
- The patient may decline life-prolonging treatment if it is futile. This is a decision that the patient or, if the patient is incompetent, his or her family should make.

- A 'do not attempt resuscitation' order is usually accepted or desired because death should be peaceful, and artificially or mechanically sustained life is of little value.

Sikhism

- Sikhs believe that everything that happens is the will of God (the Creator). The timing of birth and death should be left in the Creator's hands; therefore, Sikhs are discouraged in their faith to terminate their lives before the will of God (the Creator) dictates.

CASE HISTORIES

Cases 13.1 and 13.2 illustrate points made in this chapter.

CASE 13.1

Mrs G, a 90-year-old woman was admitted following a prolonged seizure and a urinary tract infection. She had had epilepsy for the last 4 years, moderate cognitive impairment and was registered as blind. She required assistance with her activities of daily living, provided mainly by her husband, although occasionally her daughter, who lived nearby, would help out. Mrs G's husband had had a stroke, and this affected his mobility. Mr and Mrs G had been married for 55 years.

Following initial improvement, Mrs G's condition deteriorated with a series of recurring chest and urinary infections. Her seizures became difficult to control and she was drowsy most of the time.

The consultant in charge called a meeting with the family and explained to them that Mrs G was unlikely to get back to her pre-admission condition. Mr G felt that she was suffering and said he would not like her to continue in this state. He maintained that this would have been her wish as well. In the discussion that ensued, it was agreed not to treat any further infections if they developed.

The meeting was obviously quite stressful for the family, especially for Mr G, who was quite tearful. The consultant asked if there was anything the family would like the staff to do. Mr G stated that they were devoted Roman Catholics and attended church regularly. He expressed a wish for a priest visit and to give Mrs G her last rites. This was duly arranged. The family were grateful for the fact that the medical team had considered this aspect of care and raised it with them.

CASE 13.2

An 86-year-old woman was admitted with bilateral bronchopneumonia. She had a complicated medical history of diabetes mellitus, hypertension, chronic kidney disease and spinal canal stenosis limiting her mobility.

Despite aggressive treatment she remained unwell. She became hypoxic despite oxygen therapy. Although drowsy, she remained able to take her tablets and, with help, to manage her meals.

Her breathing became laboured in the early hours of the morning of the tenth day of admission but not enough to raise the concern of the night staff. An hour later she was found dead in bed.

The night nurse contacted the son, who was the next of kin. He was told that his mother's condition had deteriorated and that he needed to come to hospital straightaway. The records show that the son asked specifically if his mother was still breathing, to which the nurse replied, 'yes', as she did not want him to drive to the hospital in a distressed state. As the son drove into the hospital, he contacted the ward to check on his mother but was then told she had passed away. He arrived at the ward in a distraught state, crying loudly and causing considerable distress to the other patients. The staff struggled to calm him down.

The son formally complained that his mother had 'started to suffer' around the time of her death and that he was unhappy with the medical care she received. Despite several letters of correspondence, the issue could not be resolved.

A meeting was arranged with the son, to go through his concerns face to face. At the meeting it was explained in detail that his mother's condition was serious and that this was conveyed to family members on at least two occasions during her hospital stay.

The son raised the point that he did not know exactly when his mother passed away. He maintained that his mother perhaps experienced an unsettled death. He felt that no attempt was made to keep her alive until he could at least arrive at her bedside. He also maintained he should have been told the previous evening so that he could have stayed by her side. He became very emotional on a couple of occasions and had to be comforted.

He was of Hindu faith and it became obvious that he was agonising over the manner of his mother's death. He firmly believed in the concept of good and bad death. His main complaint was that he was not there to comfort his mother in her last moments and to perform the religious rituals needed to send her on her way. It was acknowledged that the whole problem would not have occurred and distress to the family would have been avoided if the staff had understood the religious needs of the patient by discussing it with her and her family and agreeing on an action plan beforehand. A formal apology was expressed.

REFERENCES

1. Sulmasy DP. Spirituality, religion, and clinical care. *Chest.* 2009; **135**(6): 1634–42.
2. National Consensus Project for Quality Palliative Care. *Clinical Practice Guidelines for Quality Palliative Care.* 3rd ed. Pittsburgh, PA: National Consensus Project for Quality Palliative Care. Available at: www.nationalconsensusproject.org/NCP_Clinical_Practice_Guidelines_3rd_Edition.pdf (accessed 25 March 2014).
3. Lo B, Quill T, Tulsky J. Discussing palliative care with patients. ACP-AS1M End-of-Life Care Consensus Panel. *Ann Intern Med.* 1999; **130**(9): 744–9.
4. Musick MA, Traphagan JW, Koenig HG, *et al.* Spirituality in physical health and aging. *J Adult Dev.* 2000; **7**(2): 73–86.
5. Rosin AJ, Sonnenblick M. Autonomy and paternalism in geriatric medicine. The Jewish ethical approach to issues of feeding terminally ill patients, and to cardio-pulmonary resuscitation. *J Med Ethics.* 1998; **24**(1): 44–8.
6. Dorff EN. End-of-life: Jewish perspectives. *Lancet.* 2005; **366**(9488): 862–5.
7. Takrouri M, Halwani TM. An Islamic medical and legal prospective of do not resuscitate order in critical care medicine. *Internet J Health.* 2008; **7**(1): 1528.
8. IMANA Ethics Committee. Islamic medical ethics: the IMANA perspective. *J IMA.* 2005; **37**(1): 33–42. Available at: http://jima.imana.org/article/view/5528 (accessed 8 August 2013).
9. Sachedina A. End-of-life: the Islamic view. *Lancet.* 2005; **366**(9487): 774–9.
10. Engelhardt HT Jr, Iltis AS. End-of-life: the traditional Christian view. *Lancet.* 2005; **366**(9490): 1045–9.
11. Crawford SC. *Dilemmas of Life and Death: Hindu ethics in a North American context.* Albany, NY: State University of New York Press; 1995.
12. Desai PN. Medical ethics in India. *J Med Philos.* 1998; **13**(3): 231–55.

FURTHER READING

- Department of Health. *Spiritual Care at the End of Life: a systematic review of the literature.* London: DH; 2011. Available at: www.gov.uk/government/publications/spiritual-care-at-the-end-of-life-a-systematic-review-of-the-literature (accessed 25 March 2014).
- National Institute for Health and Care Excellence. *Quality Standard for End of Life Care for Adults: NICE quality standard 13.* London: NICE; 2011. Available at: http://publications.nice.org.uk/quality-standard-for-end-of-life-care-for-adults-qs13 (accessed 25 March 2014).
- Royal College of Physicians, National End of Life Care Programme, Association for Palliative Medicine of Great Britain and Ireland. *Improving End-of-Life Care: professional development for physicians; report of a working party.* London: RCP; 2012. Available at: www.rcplondon.ac.uk/resources/improving-end-life-care-professional-development-physicians (accessed 25 March 2014).

CHAPTER 14

Ethical issues in dementia

Gurcharan S Rai and Jim Eccles

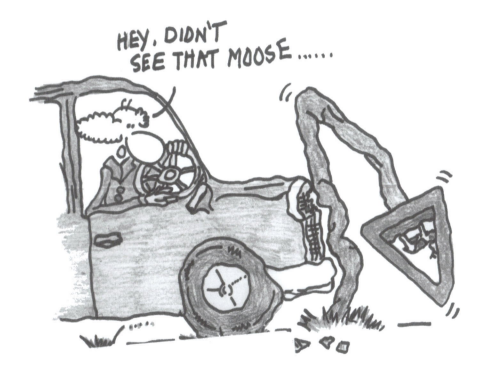

HEY, DIDN'T SEE THAT MOOSE......

INTRODUCTION

Dementia is a disease that shows increasing incidence with age. While the prevalence is about 5% in the elderly over 65 years of age, it reaches nearly 20% in those over 80 years. In clinical practice it is important to differentiate not only between acute confusional states and dementia, but also between the various types of dementia as new treatments for Alzheimer's disease become available.

Ethical issues arising in the management of dementia vary with progression of the disease. In the early stages, issues may range from questions of consent,

155

to informing the patient that he or she has a dementing illness, to decision-making capacity. In the later stages, the issues revolve around appropriate levels of care, decisions about resuscitation and end-of-life issues, financial and legal arrangements and use of restraints. Although there is no cure for dementia, new therapies are being developed to improve function and/or slow down the progression of disease. The recent introduction of acetylcholinesterase inhibitors such as donepezil, rivastigmine and galantamine has raised the ethical issue of rationing and postcode prescribing.

Over time, alteration in a patient's cognitive state may lead to a change in the doctor–patient relationship. It is not uncommon to note that a physician, after having assessed the patient, talks to the carer as if the patient were not in the room, thus ignoring the patient's feelings. It is important for us as professionals to recognise that loss of cognitive function does not mean total loss of emotions and human values. At the very least, the physician should ensure that the patient is seen on his or her own before any discussion takes place between the doctor and the carer, and any discussion that takes place should involve the patient.

ETHICAL ISSUES IN THE EARLY STAGES OF DEMENTIA

In the early stages, patients with dementia have the capacity to undertake decisions with regard to their treatment (i.e. they can choose to accept or refuse); therefore, these patients should not be treated any differently from other patients but, instead, should be allowed to exercise that choice. Denying choice compromises independence and dignity. The National Institute for Health and Care Excellence (NICE) recommends that while a person with dementia has capacity, there should be full discussion with him or her and his or her carers on the use of:

➤ advance statements on what action should be taken if the person loses the capacity to make decisions
➤ advance decisions to refuse treatment
➤ lasting power of attorney (LPA)
➤ a preferred place of care.

Informing the patient about the diagnosis

It is argued by some that because dementia is a progressive disease with no available curative treatment, some patients will be unable to accept the diagnosis, and as a result may suffer psychological distress with a subsequent reduction in hope and motivation. Although it is true that, in practice, some patients find it difficult to accept a diagnosis with a poor prognosis (e.g. they switch off during discussion), it should be possible to discuss the diagnosis sympathetically, providing support to the patient over two or more sessions. Basic principles require that we as physicians should be honest and tell the patient the truth so that the patient can exercise his or her moral and ethical right to decide, while he or she is still competent, whether the patient wishes to accept or reject treatment or investigations should he or she become incompetent. This may also lead to patients accepting the involvement of support groups or help from psychologists and community psychiatric nurses. This in turn helps through discussion to overcome psychological reactions of fear, depression and anger. In addition, patients may decide to seek guidance about advance refusals (advance directives). If there is a language barrier, the doctor should consider using independent interpreters or using written information in the preferred language and/or an accessible format.

In some cases, family members may insist that a patient should not be informed of the diagnosis. Under these circumstances it is important to clarify that a competent individual has the moral and legal right to know the diagnosis and make decisions about his or her future care, which also includes treatment.

Informing family and carers about the diagnosis

Family members may ask not only for the diagnosis to be kept from the patient but also for the diagnosis to be given to them before it is given to the patient. In the latter situation it is important to inform the family that doctors cannot, either in law or ethically, give information to a third party without the consent and agreement of a competent adult (i.e. the patient). In fact, a competent patient can ask a doctor not to talk to a particular family member, and if this happens, doctors must act in accordance with the patient's wishes. Of course in the late stages of dementia, when the patient is unlikely to have the capacity to give consent, the doctor should talk to the family. Sharing information with the family and carer involved in providing support and care to the patient will not only help the doctor to obtain insight into the patient's past wishes, but also ensure that appropriate care is organised in the best interests of the patient.

Issues surrounding genetics

Recent developments in genetics have identified mutations that predispose to Alzheimer's disease on chromosomes 21, 19, 14 and 1. The gene located on chromosome 21, an autosomal-dominant gene, was the first to be discovered in groups of families in whom the onset of dementia started at below the age of 65 years. This gene results in the production of a precursor protein B-amyloid around plaques. The second abnormal gene, located on chromosome 14 (an autosomal-dominant and a presenilin-1 gene), is responsible for 70%–80% of familial cases. The third gene locus, on chromosome 1 (presenilin 2 gene), relates to an early onset of familial dementia. Although chromosome 1 is a dominant gene, at least two examples of probable incomplete penetrance have been identified. The three disease genes responsible for familial Alzheimer's dementia (chromosomes 21, 14 and 1) account for less than 5% of all cases. Late-onset Alzheimer's dementia is a polygenic multifactorial disorder in which some gene effects may be found, but environmental and other modulatory factors may be of central importance. The gene with the greatest influence on development of late-onset dementia is called the apolipoprotein E gene and is located on chromosome 19.

Although some physicians and relatives may suggest or demand screening for families, particularly for those with familial Alzheimer's disease, the majority reject it on the grounds that there is no preventive or protective treatment currently available, and that it has the additional disadvantage of causing psychological trauma for the individual and his or her family. The Nuffield Council on Bioethics has advised against the introduction of genetic testing in disorders and diseases with multiple causes, and thus this applies to most, if not all, older patients with Alzheimer's disease. If a doctor agrees to the demand for genetic testing from a member of the family of a patient with familial Alzheimer's disease, counselling before and after testing is regarded as essential, in line with recent NICE guidance.

Ethical issues surrounding new treatment

At present there are four drugs available for use in patients with Alzheimer's disease – namely, donepezil (a piperidine-based reversible inhibitor of acetylcholinesterase), rivastigmine (a centrally selective inhibitor of acetyl-cholinesterase), galantamine (a competitive acetylcholinesterase inhibitor) and memantine (a voltage-dependent, moderate-affinity non-competitive NMDA-receptor antagonist). Donepezil, rivastigmine and galantamine are recommended for patients with moderate severity only (Mini-Mental State Examination (MMSE) score of 10–20). The revised NICE guideline recommends memantine as an option for managing Alzheimer's disease for patients who cannot take acetylcholinesterase inhibitors, and as an option for managing severe Alzheimer's disease.

In line with NICE guidelines, only specialists in the care of patients with dementia (i.e. psychiatrists, neurologists and physicians specialising in care of the elderly) are allowed to prescribe, with regular review at 6 months using the MMSE score and global, functional and behavioural assessments. Of course, the MMSE may not be appropriate as a tool for assessment for those from different ethnic groups and patients with disabilities. In these patients it is important to consider using alternative tests such as the Cambridge Cognitive Examination, the Modified Cambridge Examination for Mental Disorders of the Elderly, the Dementia Questionnaire for Mentally Retarded Persons or the Dementia Scale for Down's Syndrome. None of these drugs is curative, and not all patients with Alzheimer's disease show a response to them – between 40% and 70% of people with Alzheimer's disease benefit from acetylcholinesterase inhibitor treatment.

Although it is reasonable not to offer treatment that is deemed futile, it is ethically wrong and with the introduction of the Equality Act 2010 it would be unlawful to deny treatment to an individual on the grounds of age alone, if that treatment has been shown to be of benefit.

The other ethical issue in relation to prescribing of anti-dementia drugs is that of consent. In UK law, an adult is presumed to have the capacity to make decisions and to act upon those decisions. Therefore it follows that before an anti-dementia drug can be prescribed, a doctor must obtain the patient's consent. However, significant numbers of patients with dementia are incapable of giving consent, and if the ethical guidelines on consent to treatment are strictly adhered to, many of these patients would be wrongly deprived of treatment from which they could benefit. Therefore, it is accepted practice that if patients cannot give consent to medical treatment, the doctor should act in the patient's best interests after full consideration of the benefits and unwanted effects of the treatment, and after full consultation with the family and carers who know the patient best.

Issues surrounding patients' liberty to drive

Dementia can lead not only to changes in memory but also to impairment of judgement, visuospatial difficulties and inattentiveness. All of these changes can affect driving, and there is evidence that a diagnosis of dementia is associated with an increased risk of accidents. Patients with Alzheimer's dementia are five times more likely to have a car accident than their age-matched health controls.

What advice should doctors give to patients with dementia?

The answer to this question should be based on a full assessment of the patient, since not all patients with a diagnosis of dementia become unfit to drive at the time when the diagnosis is made. In the early stages there may not be any gross difficulties with judgement, visual perception, visuospatial discrimination or attention. Under these circumstances, patients can be advised that they may continue to drive until difficulties start to arise. However, if the patient admits to difficulties, a carer reports difficulties or the patient has a moderate degree of dementia, then that patient should be advised not to drive until a full assessment has been made. This may involve psychometric assessment by a psychologist and assessment by driver licensing authorities (such as the Driver and Vehicle Licensing Agency (DVLA) in the UK) to determine their medical fitness to hold a licence. The initial assessment by the DVLA consists of a medical enquiry about the patient addressed to his or her general practitioner regarding episodes of confusion or memory problems. In addition, they may ask for reports from consultant psychiatrists or an independent medical assessment and psychometric report. If doubt remains after this assessment, a full assessment may take place at a recognised disabled driver assessment unit, where physical and psychometric assessments are undertaken. If doubt about the person's ability to drive still persists, he or she may be asked to take a full driving test. Finally, it is important to note that simple cognitive tests such as the MMSE are very poor predictors of driving ability.

What should happen if patients continue to drive against their doctor's wishes?

It is important for us, as doctors, first to remember that we have a legal duty to respect the confidence of a patient, and second to consider not only the right of a person with dementia to maintain his or her personal freedom but also the right of everyone to be safe. Although reporting of suspected medical unfitness to drive raises an important ethical dilemma about confidentiality, most physicians now accept that the principle of confidentiality is partly or wholly balanced by a 'common good' principle for the protection of third parties. In the UK, doctors should therefore inform the DVLA in Swansea directly on failure to persuade the patient to do this him- or herself, and when the doctor has grounds to suspect that the patient is putting him- or herself or others at risk.

What is the law regarding fitness to drive?

In the UK, the Road Traffic Act 1988 and the Motor Vehicles (Driving Licences) Regulations 1996 define severe mental disorder as a relevant disability for licensing, and this includes dementia. The person is obliged by law to inform the DVLA about his or her condition. Failure to do so can result in a fine of up to £1000 and/or prosecution if the individual is involved in an accident. If a patient refuses to do this despite advice from his or her doctor and family, the doctor can inform the DVLA directly after first informing the patient of this decision.

ETHICAL PROBLEMS ASSOCIATED WITH THE LATE STAGES OF DEMENTIA

As the disease progresses, patients become increasingly less able to make decisions. However, this does not imply incompetence. Although they may not understand the benefits and risks of medical intervention, they may still be able to understand their finances or home circumstances. Therefore it is essential that competence is assessed in the area in question.

Treatment of acute illness, including decisions about resuscitation

As the disease progresses, patients become mentally incompetent and therefore unable to make decisions about treatment. Under these circumstances one should consider the following three steps under the Mental Capacity Act 2005.
1. Can the decision be delayed until the patient is capable of making the decision him- or herself? If the answer is 'yes', then the decision should be delayed; if not, then ask the following question.
2. Has the patient appointed a LPA for personal and welfare decisions, or made a valid advance decision?
3. If the answer to question 2 is 'no', then the patient's best interests should be treated using the best interests checklist (*see* Table 14.1).

In an emergency where formal capacity assessment is not possible, immediate treatment can be administered on the basis of assumed consent in a cooperating patient or in his or her best interests until the patient's condition has been stabilised, at which stage best interests assessment can be performed.

In reality, the clinical decision-making process may involve looking at the benefits as well as the risks, burdens and side effects of treatment, and the patient's quality of life. Since quality of life is difficult to assess, it becomes increasingly necessary to make a judgement based on the severity and prognosis of the disease. If the patient is clearly nearing the end of life, it becomes both reasonable and acceptable not to attempt any futile treatment that could offer the false hope of artificially prolonging that life. Symptomatic treatments such as antipyretics for fever, oral care, bowel care to prevent constipation, bladder care to prevent retention of urine, and skin care to prevent pressure sores all become increasingly important in patients nearing the end of life. As death becomes imminent, the priorities are symptom relief and personal dignity, and in this situation cardiopulmonary resuscitation should not be attempted. Quite apart from being futile, attempts to revive a patient at such a late stage would also deprive both the patient and the family of privacy and dignity at the end of a long illness.

TABLE 14.1 Checklist for determining the patient's best interests

Factors to be taken into account when making a 'best interests' assessment

- Identifying things that an individual would take into account if acting for him- or herself
- The patient's past and present expressed wishes
- The patient's beliefs and values
- Views of family, friends, carers and general practitioner regarding what the patient would have wanted for him- or herself
- Views of an independent mental capacity advocate if the patient has no family or friends

Percutaneous endoscopic gastrostomy feeding

CASE 14.1

An 85-year-old woman who has severe Alzheimer's disease is admitted to hospital from a nursing home with right lower lobe pneumonia. Assessment by a speech and language therapist reveals poor swallowing on admission to hospital. Nurses start her on nasogastric feeding. During the next 7 days the patient pulls out the nasogastric tube on six occasions. After those 7 days, when her clinical features of pneumonia have improved, the question of percutaneous endoscopic gastrostomy (PEG) is raised. The speech and language therapist feels that the patient is unlikely to pull out her PEG tube, as it does not normally cause discomfort.

Swallowing problems are not uncommon in patients with dementia with the progression of disease, and particularly at times of acute illness. In some the ability to swallow returns, while in others the swallowing difficulties remain, making oral intake unsafe. At this stage PEG may be considered and discussed as a long-term option between the members of the multidisciplinary team and the family. Often the question of whether it is appropriate to place a PEG tube in a severely demented patient will be asked.

In such situations, the doctor should consider the following points.

➤ The benefits and risks associated with PEG in this group of patients. One large influential review failed to find any evidence that tube feeding patients with advanced dementia prolongs survival, prevents aspiration pneumonia, reduces the risk of pressure sores or improves physical function and comfort. In addition, PEG is associated with local irritation, which can lead to potentially fatal complications, such as infection and haemorrhage.

➤ The benefits and risks associated with PEG in the patient concerned. Co-morbidity in an individual increases the risk of complications and mortality.

➤ Whether the patient has left instructions in the form of a valid and applicable advance decision. Enquiry should also be made as to whether the patient has appointed an attorney, using the LPA, to cover medical treatment.

If the patient has not made an advance refusal or appointed an attorney to decide about medical treatment, then the decision should be made in the patient's best interests, using the assessment recommended by the Mental Capacity Act 2005, including the following points.

➤ Discussion of the benefits and risks of PEG feeding with family, carers and staff involved in caring for the patient. An independent mental capacity advocate should be appointed if there are no suitable relatives or close friends to consult.

➤ Assessment of the patient's present behaviour. Is the patient trying to indicate that he or she does not wish to be fed, by pulling out nasogastric tubes repeatedly, or by declining to take food orally when it is offered? Alternatively, does the patient demonstrate signs of hunger, and a desire to try foods that may be deemed as unsuitable because of swallowing difficulties?

In some patients with dementia, dysphagia may not be due to the dementia itself but may be the result of another physical condition. Under those circumstances it would be more appropriate to consider PEG feeding. However, if the decline in nutritional intake is due to the dementia itself, then the disease has reached a very advanced stage, and a more palliative approach to care may be indicated. The NICE and Social Care Institute for Excellence guidance recommends that tube feeding is not usually appropriate for patients with severe dementia who are nearing the end of life.

Use of physical and chemical restraints

Personality and behavioural changes are common with progression of the disease process. Aberrant behaviour with or without wandering, particularly in the presence of an acute illness, may become a major problem for the patient's family or carer, as well as for those professionals who are providing help and care for those affected by the disease. Although to restrain someone physically or chemically just for the benefit of carers or hospital staff would be wrong, it may be considered where it is in the best interests of the patient. Section 6 of the Mental Capacity Act 2005 defines 'restraint' as the use or threat of force when an incapacitated person resists. The Mental Capacity Act 2005 permits the use of such restraint if it is both justifiable, because it is necessary to prevent harm to the incapacitated person, and proportionate to the likelihood and seriousness of that harm. One should also include the caregiver's views in the decision-making process about any possible restraint (*see* Chapter 15, 'The lawful use of restraints').

The ethical guidelines on restraint proposed by the Ethics and Humanities Subcommittee of the American Academy of Neurology included the following points.

➤ Restraints should only be ordered when they contribute to the safety of the patient or others and are not simply a convenience for the staff.

➤ Restraints should not be ordered as a substitute for careful evaluation and surveillance of the patient, as appropriate for good medical practice.

➤ The perceived need for restraints should trigger medical assessment and investigation of the precise reason for them, intended to correct the underlying medical or psychological problem.

➤ If a proxy decision-maker is known, restraints should only be ordered after full discussion of the risks and benefits. However, in an acute situation doctors should act in the best interests of the patient.

➤ When they are indicated, pharmacological agents should be used at the lowest dose possible.

➤ All restraints should be reassessed frequently so that they may be in effect for the shortest duration necessary to achieve their goals.

Use of monitoring equipment

Assistive technology continues to develop not only in order to enable independence for the elderly but also for the purpose of monitoring the well-being of an individual. Video and electronic tags are now widely available and are being employed by some institutions and private homes for monitoring elderly patients with dementia, who have a tendency to wander and a predisposition to fall. There is no doubt that the use of such equipment raises issues such as freedom and liberty, and it is therefore important that any decision to use them takes into account such important issues and places the individual older person at the centre of the decision-making process. The final decision should be based on the principle of 'best interests' of the older person, and not on the interest of the staff or carer or the home itself.

Law and financial handling capacity of patients with dementia

As dementia progresses, patients become increasingly less able to handle their financial affairs. In the early stages, an individual may ask another person to help collect a pension or pay bills on the odd occasion. However, for permanent arrangements the patient with dementia who has the capacity to understand and make decisions should be advised to make a LPA in line with the Mental Capacity Act 2005.

The LPA covers property and financial affairs as well as personal welfare covering social and medical care. To be effective, a LPA will have to be registered with the Office of the Public Guardian.

In financial matters, a LPA gives 'general' authority to carry out all transactions on behalf of the individual, or specific authority. This gives the person authority to sign cheques or withdraw money from the bank.

When there is no LPA, the Court of Protection can be asked to appoint a deputy who will be able to take decisions on financial matters as authorised by the court. Although the deputy can also be given authority to act on social and health matters, he or she will not have authority to refuse consent to life-sustaining treatment.

What about those who neglect themselves at home because of dementia but refuse to accept help?

In the late stages of dementia, personal neglect is not only common but also often denied by the patient. Commonly this information becomes available when a person is admitted to hospital with an acute illness. A dilemma arises, with conflict between autonomy and beneficence, when the patient recovers from the physical illness and insists on going home. The individual's wishes (patient's autonomy) must be respected. Actions must be taken to reduce or minimise neglect as far as possible through discussion with the patient, his or her family and carers, and all of the agencies involved in providing community services. If this is not possible, and the patient refuses to accept help or to leave home to go into a safer environment, and from assessment it is clear that the patient is unable to understand the risks of going home, then a decision should be taken in the patient's best interests. Even then, the Mental Capacity Act 2005 encourages us to consider the patient's wishes and to choose the 'least restrictive option'. In a wide-ranging report on ethical issues in the care of people with dementia, the Nuffield Council on Bioethics recommended that the concept of risk assessment in such situations should be replaced by a more balanced risk–benefit assessment, to ensure that people with dementia are not unreasonably denied the opportunity to maintain their independence.

In the UK, 'guardianship' under the Mental Health Act 1983 can be exercised in order to ensure the welfare of the patient and the protection of others. This will allow the patient to be moved to a safer environment. To enforce this section, the signatures of two registered practitioners (one of whom should be a mental health specialist) are required. The other sections of the Mental Health Act 1983 can also be used to detain patients with dementia. For example, under section 4 a person can be admitted as an emergency if the relatives and social workers cannot cope with the patient's behaviour. The period of detention under the section is a maximum of 72 hours, but this can be changed to 28 days by seeking a specialist opinion.

Section 47 of the National Assistance Act 1948 can also be used to admit a person to hospital who is unable to care for him- or herself at home, is not receiving care at home, is suffering from a grave chronic disease or is living in unsanitary conditions. This Act does not allow treatment to be given against the patient's wishes. The other drawback is that, unlike the Mental Health Act 1983, it does not provide safeguards for the person with respect to review procedures.

The revised Mental Health Act 2007 has amended the Mental Capacity Act 2005 to include new safeguards to prevent the casual 'deprivation of liberty' in the care of people with impaired mental capacity. These new safeguards, which were implemented on 1 April 2009, will have a significant impact on the arrangements for the long-term care of such patients, and they may also apply in the case of patients who need to be restrained while in hospital. They will require that a series of formal assessments of mental health, capacity and best interests are undertaken before the deprivation of liberty can be authorised. Although the Mental Health Act 2007 has not resulted in section 47 of the National Assistance Act 1948 being repealed, it is clear that in cases where the new 'deprivation of liberty' safeguards are already in operation, they will take precedence. According to the wording of the Mental Health Act 2007, there would appear to be no reason why the new safeguards will not apply following an admission under section 47, but this may ultimately need to be clarified by case law.

Abuse of the elderly with dementia

Mental impairment makes the elderly vulnerable to abuse, which may take the form of physical, mental and financial abuse as well as deprivation of nutrition, help in activities of daily living and prescribed drugs. Recognition of abuse can be difficult because physical changes may mimic the changes of ageing and the elderly person may be unwilling or unable to admit to abuse. Action against suspected abuse in an institution may be possible through statutory bodies that visit institutions and action against individuals who ill-treat or neglect a person who lacks capacity is possible using the Mental Capacity Act 2005, which has introduced this as a criminal offence that carries a penalty of imprisonment for a term of up to 5 years.

In the case of a person who is being abused and still has capacity, it is difficult to take action against a relative or carer who is suspected of abuse if the elderly person is unable or unwilling to cooperate. This raises the important ethical issue of whether action should be taken against the wishes of an elderly person in order to protect him or her. Unfortunately, there is no law that allows professionals to make the elderly wards of court, as is the case with children. Therefore, we may have no option but to continue to work closely with all of the carers involved in providing care for the older person, including relatives who may themselves be the abusers of an elderly patient. It is hoped that vigilant and consistent contact will reduce the likelihood of abuse. Local health authorities and social services have drawn up guidelines for staff to follow, and all cases of possible abuse should be reported to the multi-agency safeguarding authorities.

KEY POINTS

- In the early stages, patients with dementia have the full capacity to undertake decision-making with regard to their treatment, and therefore they should not be treated differently from other patients.
- Basic principles require the physician to tell the patient that he or she has dementia.
- Since there are no available preventive or therapeutic agents that can cure dementia, it is not yet necessary to carry out genetic testing of a family member.
- Any new effective treatment that is developed should be available for patients, and no one should be denied treatment solely on the grounds of age. Any rationing should be open to public scrutiny.
- Patients with obvious impairment of judgement or visuospatial difficulties should be asked to stop driving. If they fail to take this advice, they should be reported to the Driver and Vehicle Licensing Agency, even if it means breaking the rule about patient confidentiality.
- In the late stages of disease, doctors may have to make decisions about which treatment is best for the individual. Assessment of best interests should be performed in line with the Mental Capacity Act 2005.
- In end-stage dementia, artificial tube feeding is not usually appropriate, and palliative care should be available when required.
- Restraint should only be used if it contributes to the safety of the patient or others, and it should not be used for the convenience of staff.
- In the early stages of dementia, patients should be encouraged to consider appointing a lasting power of attorney and making a valid advance decision.
- Patients who neglect themselves may still need to be admitted to hospital under section 47 of the National Assistance Act 1948, or moved into a residential home using guardianship under the Mental Health Act 1983.
- New safeguards to prevent the deprivation of liberty are widely applicable to the care of patients with impaired mental capacity.

FURTHER READING

- American Academy of Neurology Ethics and Humanities Subcommittee. Ethical issues in the management of the demented patient. *Neurology*. 1996; **46**(4): 1180–3.
- Department for Constitutional Affairs. *Mental Capacity Act 2005 Code of Practice*. London: TSO; 2007. Available at: www.justice.gov.uk/downloads/protecting-the-vulnerable/mca/mca-code-practice-0509.pdf (accessed 26 March 2014).
- Department of Health. *Reference Guide to the Mental Health Act 1983*. London: DH; 2008.
- Finucane TE, Christmas C, Travis K. Tube feeding in patients with advanced dementia: a review of the evidence. *JAMA*. 1999; **282**(14): 1365–70
- Government Equalities Office. *Equality Act Guidance*. London: GEO; 2010. Available at:

www.gov.uk/government/publications/equality-act-guidance (accessed 6 November 2013).

- Harris J. It's not NICE to discriminate. *J Med Ethics*. 2005; **31**(7): 373–5.
- Ministry of Justice. *Deprivation of Liberty Safeguards: code of practice*. London: Ministry of Justice; 2008.
- National Institute for Health and Clinical Excellence. *Donepezil, galantamine, rivastigmine and memantine for the treatment of Alzheimer's disease (review)*. NICE technology appraisal guidance 111. London: NICE; 2007. Available at www.nice.org.uk/guidance/index.jsp?action=article&o=51047 (accessed 6 November 2013).
- National Institute for Health and Clinical Excellence. *Donepezil, galantamine, rivastigmine and memantine for the treatment of Alzheimer's disease: review of NICE technology appraisal guidance 111*. NICE technology appraisal guidance 217. London: NICE; 2011. Available at: www.nice.org.uk/guidance/TA217 (accessed 6 November 2013)
- National Institute for Health and Clinical Excellence; Social Care Institute for Excellence. *Dementia: supporting people with dementia and their carers in health and social care*. NICE clinical guideline 42. London: NICE; 2006. Available at: http://guidance.nice.org.uk/CG42 (accessed 6 November 2013).
- Nuffield Council on Bioethics. *Dementia: ethical issues*. London: Nuffield Council on Bioethics; 2009.
- Post SG. Alzheimer's disease: ethics and the progression of dementia. *Clin Geriatr Med*. 1994; **10**(2): 379–94.
- Post SG, Whitehouse PJ. Fairhill Guidelines on ethics of the care of people with Alzheimer's disease: a clinical summary. *J Am Geriatr Soc*. 1995; **43**(12): 1423–9.

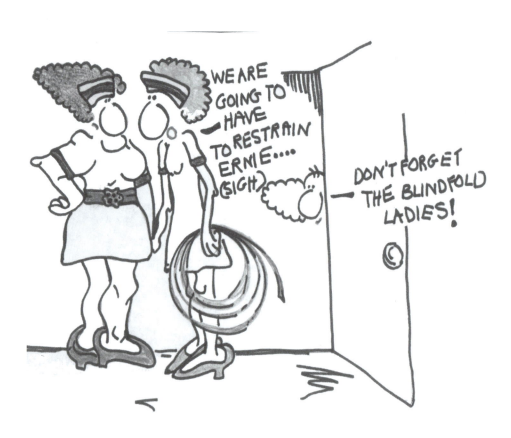

CHAPTER 15

The lawful use of restraints

Gwen M Sayers and Gurcharan S Rai

INTRODUCTION

Restraining a competent person without consent is unlawful and constitutes a criminal assault; therefore, restraining one who lacks capacity to consent requires sound justification. Restraining individuals reduces their autonomy and limits their choices. They are prevented from pursuing their own good in their own manner. However, despite this, John Stuart Mill, who so described this fundamental freedom in his essay 'On Liberty',[1] accorded it only to competent individuals rather than those who, in the care of others, required protection from injury to themselves and injury to others.

CASE 15.1

Mrs A, an 86-year-old woman with dementia, is admitted to a general medical ward with pneumonia that is successfully treated. Although she has recovered, her discharge is delayed because she is unable to care for herself. While awaiting institutional placement, her behaviour becomes problematic. She tends to sleep during the day and is noisy and aggressive at night, when she wanders and climbs into other patients' beds. There are fewer nurses on the night shift and they struggle to provide the amount of supervision required by Mrs A. They therefore ask the doctors to prescribe night-time sedation. The sedation is cumulative and the patient now sleeps both day and night. Consequently her food and fluid intake declines. One morning she is unable to be aroused. Blood tests show that the serum sodium level is 181 mmol/L. Although she is treated with intravenous fluids, she dies soon after without regaining consciousness.

There is evidence that the use of restraints increases in direct proportion to the age of the patient and the level of cognitive impairment, regardless of the setting.[2] Restraint may be physical or chemical, but the underlying assumptions are those articulated by Mill – confused patients are restrained for their own benefit or the benefit of others. The flip side of these benefits is the damage that is undoubtedly caused by restraint, both by reducing the dignity of patients and by exposing them to the risk of adverse physical effects. Hence, as in other areas of ethics, before deciding to restrain a patient a benefit–burden equation needs to be balanced. Furthermore, the way in which the equation is balanced should be compatible with recent changes in English law.

There are good moral arguments supporting aversion to restraint. Dodds[3] argues that respect for autonomy is a duty that persists, and is thus owed even to those who lack legal capacity. She therefore believes that there is only limited justification for restraining patients on paternalistic grounds.[3] There are equally sound clinical reasons to avoid restraining frail elderly people, because of risks associated with their use (*see* Box 15.1).

BOX 15.1 Risks associated with use of restraints

Injuries from falls	Accidental death from strangulation
Decline in function	Skin breakdown
Cardiac stress	Reduced appetite
Dehydration	Emotional and behavioural problems

Source: Evans and Strumpf[2]

Although restraint has been curtailed since 1987 in the United States – by the Nursing Home Reform Act of 1987 as part of the Omnibus Budget Reconciliation Act of 1987 – in the UK the Care Standards Act 2000, the Care Homes Regulations 2001 and the Domiciliary Care Agencies Regulations 2002 do not prohibit the use of restraint. For example, regulation 13 (7) of the Care Homes Regulations 2001 states:

> The registered person shall ensure that no service user is subject to physical restraint unless restraint of the kind employed is the only practicable means of securing the welfare of that or any other service user and there are exceptional circumstances.

Furthermore, regulation 13 (8) states:

> On any occasion on which a service user is subject to physical restraint, the registered person should record the circumstances, including the nature of the restraint.

The question of when, if ever, to restrain a confused elderly patient is therefore arguable. This chapter will outline situations where restraint may be necessary – when the benefits outweigh the harms – and will describe safeguards to ensure that restraint is proportionate and justified. The Human Rights Act 1998 (HRA) and the Mental Capacity Act 2005 (MCA) will be used to support an approach regarding whether and when restraint is lawful.

THE USE OF RESTRAINT

Elderly patients in hospital wards and nursing homes are in an unfamiliar environment shared with strangers. They may be prone to disorientation, which can manifest as disturbed behaviour, especially if they are cognitively impaired, acutely ill or on medication. Discomfort (due to pain, constipation or a full bladder) may cause attempts to wander, or boredom may prompt a wish to escape. Many of these patients may be unsteady, have poor vision and be likely to fall. Falls can result in serious injuries – notably, fractured hips and subdural haematomata, either of which can cause death. Therefore staff, afraid of being charged with a breach of their duty of care, may use restraint as a defensive measure.

Three main types of restraint are used within an institutional setting.

1. *Restraints that limit mobility*. Restraints that prevent free mobility include bedrails that hinder patients trying to leave the bed, and chairs with trays that entrap patients in a seated position. Bedrails, however, are not necessarily a deterrent to patients determined to climb out of bed. If a confused patient manages to scale them, the rails increase the height of the fall, thereby increasing the damage sustained. All forms of restraint resulting in immobility take their toll by causing loss of muscle strength and a predisposition towards the development of pressure sores. Therefore, measures implemented to protect the patient from the risk of falling may lead to greater, although different, dangers.

2. *Restraints that prevent access to one's body*. Restraints that prevent patients from accessing their own bodies include tying patients' limbs or using mittens. Such restraints are used to facilitate the administration of medication, to prevent patients dislodging nasogastric tubes and other internal lines, or to prevent self-harm. These restraints are now rarely used, both because they are degrading and because of their potential adverse effects. Patients may struggle against ties, resulting in abrasive skin injuries or even gangrene of a limb through disruption of blood supply.

3. *Chemical restraints*. Chemical restraints or sedating agents are used, especially on general wards, to contain noisy and disruptive patients or those with behavioural problems – largely for the sake of other patients. The use of major tranquillisers for patients suffering from dementia has been broadly condemned because of adverse effects. Apart from over-sedation as described in Case 15.1, these drugs have also been linked to increased cardiovascular mortality. Their other common side effects, such as postural hypotension and extrapyramidal manifestations, increase the likelihood of falls. Moreover, these drugs can worsen confusional states, so magnifying the problem for which they were initially prescribed.

There is thus good reason to advocate zero tolerance of restraints. This ideal, however, would require resources in excess of those available within the National Health Service. For example, disruptive and aggressive patients nursed in side rooms with one-to-one care would not require sedating agents. Patients with internal lines would not dislodge them if watched constantly and discouraged from handling their tubes. Patients would not fall out of bed if nursed in a side room on a mattress placed on the floor.

Such measures are usually not possible because, except in intensive care settings or in psychiatric wards, the nurse-to-patient ratio makes close monitoring of all confused patients difficult if not impossible, especially at night. Side rooms are a scarce commodity that may be prioritised for patients with infectious diseases or dying patients who require privacy. The best alternative to prohibition of restraint is to adopt a high threshold to the use of restraint and develop a policy that ensures reasonable safeguards and appropriate justification for those cases where restraint appears to be the only safe option. The policy would have to comply with recent UK legislation.[4]

HUMAN RIGHTS ACT 1998

The HRA, which came into effect in 2000, made it unlawful for a public authority to act in a way that was incompatible with any of the articles incorporated in the European Convention on Human Rights. The term 'public authority' encompasses National Health Service trusts as well as individual doctors who, in the course of their duties, treat patients within the remit of the trusts. The articles relevant to restraint that will be considered are articles 2, 3 and 8. Article 5 (the right to liberty), which applies to individuals who are detained, falls outside the scope of this chapter.

Article 2: the right to life

Article 2 imposes a strong duty on the state not to interfere with life, and a weaker duty to protect life. This implies a strict prohibition against causing death, without a correspondingly stringent obligation to preserve life at all costs. The European Court of Human Rights, by recognising a limitation on the obligation to preserve life, released authorities from an impossible or disproportionate burden.

This approach is echoed in common law and in guidance provided by the General Medical Council and the British Medical Association. Doctors are obliged to provide life-prolonging treatment only when it is in the patient's best interests. Therefore, if continuing treatment is considered to be in an incompetent patient's best interests and the patient's life will be threatened if restraints are not used, the doctor may be obliged to restrain the patient in order to provide life-prolonging treatment.

CASE 15.2

Mr B, an acutely confused elderly man, has developed *Clostridium difficile* infection following treatment of a urinary tract infection. He has profuse diarrhoea and requires medication and hydration. However, Mr B refuses oral intake and pulls out both nasogastric tubes and intravenous lines. His wife asks whether his hands can be immobilised so that treatment can be effectively administered in order to save his life. This is accomplished by using mittens. After a few days of treatment his confusional state improves, the mittens are removed and oral fluids and medications are resumed. He is discharged home when well.

When treatment is both life-prolonging and in the patient's best interests, there would need to be strong justification for not using restraints if restraints are essential for treatment. This is when article 3 rights may be relevant.

Article 3: prohibition of torture

Sometimes two articles of the HRA, like two moral principles, can conflict. For example, we cannot always respect an individual patient's confidentiality when doing so threatens public interests. So it is with articles 2 and 3. Although article 2 confers a right to life, this right is not absolute. There are times when the nature of life-prolonging treatment may be disproportionately painful, or pointless if the benefits to be gained are short term. In such cases treatment, particularly if it requires restraint, may be at odds with article 3 rights.

The full text of article 3 is: 'No-one should be subjected to inhuman or degrading treatment or punishment'. On this basis, there could be argument for a blanket prohibition on restraint, so allowing article 3 rights always to trump those conferred by article 2. However, restraint, when necessary medically and used in conformity with medical standards, has been deemed legally acceptable by the European Court of Human Rights; but the type of restraint, and the way in which it is used, can breach article 2 rights. Furthermore, denial of treatment has, in itself, been found to amount to degrading treatment by the European Court.

In the UK this ruling is echoed in common law. In the case of *Re MB (Medical Treatment)*,[5] Butler-Sloss LJ said that, when treating an incompetent patient, doctors needed to judge in each case the degree of force or compulsion necessary. They had to balance whether to continue or discontinue forcibly imposed treatment.

Article 8: the right to respect for private and family life

Article 8 rights cover the individual's physical integrity. This becomes particularly important when conflict arises between the relatives and the health professionals. In *Glass v United Kingdom*,[6] doctors withheld resuscitation and administered morphine to a severely disabled child, despite the mother's objections and without judicial authorisation. This treatment was found to breach article 8 by interfering with the child's right to respect for physical integrity. The court did not consider the issue of whether the mother had article 8 rights separate from those of the patient.

Thus, human rights law informs us that restraint, although degrading at face value, is acceptable when used (proportionately) in order to treat a patient who would otherwise have to forego beneficial treatment. This only applies when treatment provides a significant benefit, such as life prolongation, or when it prevents a significant harm. It must be borne in mind that failure to treat in such cases may also be degrading. In the case of individuals who are not competent, the decision regarding treatment or withholding treatment should be discussed with relatives, and when disagreement arises (particularly in the case of minors) there may be need for judicial review.

MENTAL CAPACITY ACT 2005

Whereas the HRA provides a broad-brush approach to rights and freedoms, the MCA, which came into force in 2007, is more specific in its directives. Prior to the MCA, in English law no person could provide or withhold proxy consent for an incompetent adult. Instead, doctors were authorised to treat such patients in their best interests on the basis of necessity. Therefore, in the case of restraints used to administer life-saving treatment, the clinical team would be authorised to make the decision, as described earlier in the case of *Re MB (Medical Treatment)*. The MCA changes this by allowing a donor (the patient) to confer a lasting power of attorney on a donee, with authority to make decisions concerning the patient's personal welfare.

Section 6 of the MCA defines restraint as either the use or threat of use of force in order to undertake an action that the patient resists, or restriction of the patient's freedom of movement, whether or not the patient resists. Section 11 of the Act further imposes restrictions on the lasting power of attorney when it comes to restraint by requiring three conditions to be satisfied.

1. The patient must lack capacity in relation to the matter in question.
2. The donee must believe that the restraining act is necessary to prevent harm to the patient.
3. The restraint must be a proportionate response to the likelihood of harm to the patient and the seriousness of the harm.

The MCA requires that all decisions made on behalf of incompetent people must be made in their best interests and takes a significant step towards empowering proxy decision-makers to choose what constitutes the best interests of their loved ones. If there is no donee with lasting power of attorney, the MCA requires the clinical decision-maker to take into account the views of anyone engaged in caring for the person, provided it is practical and appropriate to consult them. Therefore, it is good practice to consult relatives whenever feasible before using restraints.

CASE 15.3

Mrs C, a patient in her nineties who has dementia, is admitted to hospital with a fractured hip following a fall at the nursing home where she lives. She requires sedation in order to X-ray her hip and she resists all attempts to draw blood or insert lines. The orthopaedic surgeon says that she is unlikely to survive an operation and recommends pain palliation. Her relatives believe that Mrs C has no quality of life and that surgery would be cruel. They say that she would refuse surgery if she were capable of deciding. Although able to swallow, Mrs C refuses food, fluids and oral medication. Restraining her in order to hydrate or nourish her is not thought to be in her best interests, since her prospects for recovery are negligible. She is treated with pain-relieving patches and dies peacefully within a few days.

GUIDELINES REGARDING RESTRAINT

All hospitals and nursing homes should have policies regarding restraint. When deciding whether or not to restrain a patient, the following factors should be considered.
- Restraining a competent patient without his or her consent is unlawful.
- When an incompetent patient requires medical treatment that can only be administered by using restraint, this is permissible provided:
  - the form of restrain used is the least restrictive possible and used for the shortest time possible
  - the treatment proposed must be in the patient's best interests
  - the consequences of not treating will be seriously harmful to the patient
  - restraint should be a short-term measure with the expectation of recovery
  - restraint is practically possible.
- When an incompetent patient cannot be safely nursed without restraint, this is permissible provided:
  - the form of restraint used is the least restrictive possible and used for the shortest time possible
  - all other avenues of nursing without restraint have been explored
  - not restraining the patient will pose a serious threat to the safety of the patient or of others.
- In all cases where restraint is deemed necessary, assent should be sought from relatives. If the relatives refuse assent to restraint in order to administer life-prolonging treatment that the medical team believe is in the patient's best interests, a legal opinion should be sought.
- In all cases where restraint is believed to be necessary, the reasons why restraint is used and with whom it was discussed should be carefully documented in the patient's notes.

KEY POINTS

- Restraining a competent person without consent is unlawful and constitutes a criminal assault.
- The Human Rights Act 1998 and the Mental Capacity Act 2005 are relevant to the use of restraints for patients who lack capacity to consent.
- Human rights law informs us that restraint, although degrading at face value, is acceptable when used (proportionately) in order to treat a patient who would otherwise have to forego beneficial treatment.
- Restraint, when medically necessary and used in conformity with medical standards, has been found to be legally acceptable by the European Court of Human Rights.
- Denial of treatment can also amount to degrading treatment in law.
- Section 6 of the Mental Capacity Act 2005 sets limitations on acts that involve restraint. Section 11 of the Act places restrictions on those with lasting powers of attorney who restrain, or authorise restraint of, a patient who lacks capacity.
- All hospitals and nursing homes should have policies regarding the use of restraints.

REFERENCES

1. Mill JS. *Three Essays: On liberty; Representative government; The subjection of women.* Oxford: Oxford University Press; 1975.
2. Evans LK, Strumpf NE. Tying down the elderly: a review of the literature on physical restraint. *J Am Geriatr Soc.* 1989; **37**(1): 65–74.
3. Dodds S. Exercising restraint: autonomy, welfare and elderly patients. *J Med Ethics.* 1996; **22**(3): 160–3.
4. Sayers GM, Gabe SM. Restraint in order to feed: justifying a lawful policy for the UK. *Eur J Health Law.* 2007; **14**(1): 3–20.
5. *Re MB (Medical Treatment)* [1997] 2 FLR 426.
6. *Glass v United Kingdom* (2004) Application no. 61827/00.

CHAPTER 16

Quality of life in healthcare decisions

Ann Bowling

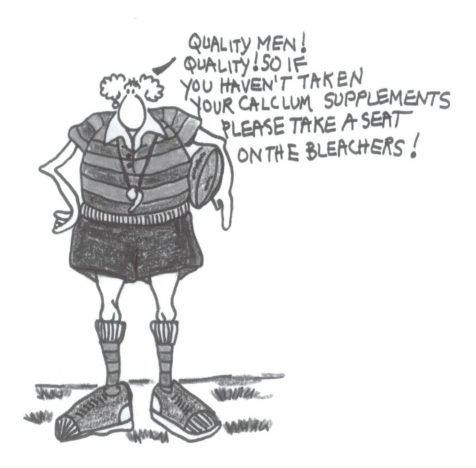

INTRODUCTION: QUALITY OF LIFE VERSUS LENGTH OF LIFE

Research in the United States indicates that patients have expressed a preference for survival for a shorter life of improved quality.[1,2] However, research on cancer patients in the UK has shown that most patients would accept toxic chemotherapy for minimal benefit in relation to prolongation of life.[3] Similarly, newly admitted inpatients under and over the age of 65, with acute coronary syndrome, reported that they would accept any treatment, however extreme, to return to their former health.[4] Research in the United States has also shown that most patients in geriatric wards indicated that they wanted to be resuscitated if their heart stopped beating, while few of their doctors had marked them for resuscitation in the medical notes.[5] It appears that doctors often rate the quality of life of the patient as lower than the patient perceives it, and the life itself of lower value than the patient rates it. The only way to face ethical dilemmas about treatments is to ask the patient about his or her perception of his or her quality of life and about his or her treatment preferences.

AGE-RELATED TREATMENT POLICIES

Negative assumptions about the quality of life of elderly people, together with a general ageism in Western society, have led to age cut-off points for treatments, which are not based on the evidence of clinical effectiveness, in some health districts. This is apparent, for example, in cardiology in relation to access to rehabilitation centres, cardiological investigations and specific, clinically effective treatments (e.g. revascularisation through coronary artery bypass graft (CABG)).[6,7]

However, increasingly the literature on health-related quality of life does not justify age-related policies. For example, a 5-year follow-up study of the broader quality of life of 1371 patients aged over 74 years at operation (mean age at operation, 77 years) and 257 'neutral-risk' patients (mean age at operation, 58 years), all of whom were undergoing CABG, reported that CABG is justified in very elderly people because the health-related quality of the extended survival was as good as that reported for younger patients and that for age-adjusted populations.[8] Although few clinical trials of treatments currently include patients aged over 65 or 70 years, it is important to measure the effects of treatments in older people as well as in younger subjects. This is more pertinent with the ageing of the population, and evidence of a healthier older population than in the past, together with the emphasis on positive ageing and equal rights to appropriate and clinically effective treatments among all age groups.

Although over-investigation and medical intervention to prolong life at the expense of quality of life at any age merit ethical debate, and while any mortality risk must be balanced against the potential gains in life years and in quality of life, it is important to ensure equal access to clinically effective and appropriate treatments from which older as well as younger people can benefit in the broadest sense.

MEASURING HEALTH-RELATED QUALITY OF LIFE

Such studies indicate the value of measuring health-related quality of life when assessing the outcome of clinical interventions. The broader measurement of health outcome has become a cornerstone of health services research. Purchasers of healthcare want to know what health gain interventions provide. This emphasis is positive, and health-related quality-of-life assessment is increasingly incorporated into criteria for the assessment of people's needs for effective services. Treatments and interventions need to be evaluated in terms of whether they are more likely to lead to an outcome of a life worth living in social, psychological and physical terms, and people themselves are the best judges of this in relation to their own lives.

Health-related quality of life is a subjective concept, and relates to the perceived effects of health status on the ability to live a fulfilling life. This encompasses functional ability in relation to ability to perform self-care tasks, domestic tasks and mobility, role functioning (e.g. ability to function in work, social roles such as parenting, and so forth), the existence and quality of relationships and social interaction, psychological well-being (e.g. life satisfaction, adjustment, coping ability), autonomy and control, and mental health (e.g. anxiety, depression, cognitive state). As with the concept, the potential range of dimensions of health-related quality of life that could be measured in studies of health outcomes is wide. A population survey of people aged 65 years that asked them how they perceived quality of life reported that they emphasised psychological characteristics (e.g. outlook on life), health and functional ability, social relationships, neighbourhood (e.g. safety, facilities, transport), having enough money and retaining their independence.[9] Individualised measures are more complex to analyse than standardised questionnaires and scales, but they are invaluable where there is uncertainty about whether all relevant questions have been included in a questionnaire, and for informing the items (questions) that make up scales and enhancing their content validity. For example, respondents' detailed statements about quality of life in the former study were used to form Likert scale ('Strongly agree' to 'Strongly disagree') statements for the multidimensional Older People's Quality of Life Questionnaire, which the author is currently testing with three national samples of older people, and with good results to date.

On a day-to-day basis, quality of life on the ward may have to be based on subjective assessment, taking into account what the patient thinks, and his or her morale, ability to communicate, mental capacity, degree of incontinence and physical dependency. For example, a person with end-stage dementia who cannot recognise his or her loved ones can be assumed to have reached a stage where, to that person, the meaning of human life has deteriorated, and he or she therefore has a poor quality of life.

As Elder[10] pointed out, common justifications for inequitable treatment of older people are perceived lack of benefit, the belief that treatments for older people represent an inappropriate use of scarce resources and the misconception that patients do not want more invasive treatments. He argued that clinicians do not need to know if an older person will benefit more or less than a younger person from a specific treatment, but rather whether a patient of any age will benefit more from a specific treatment than from usual care. The justification of inequity with reference to the appropriate use of resources by age of patient has been reinforced by health policy decisions (e.g. the UK's National Institute for Health and Care Excellence) using quality-adjusted life years, which are inherently ageist.

CHOOSING A MEASURE OF HEALTH-RELATED QUALITY OF LIFE

When choosing a health-related quality-of-life measure, or a battery of measures, key questions to consider are whether a generic or disease-specific measure is needed, and whether this should be supplemented with more detailed, domain-specific measures (e.g. depression scales) that are important to the aims of the study. The type of scale and domain-specific scales will vary according to the type of patient under study.

Generic measures usually tap social, psychological and physical areas of life. They are used for population health profiles and in order to make comparisons with other conditions (e.g. outcome of treatments for different conditions). The latter are useful when comparisons of the costs of treatments in relation to their benefits (outcomes) are required.

POPULAR MEASUREMENT SCALES

One of the most popular, concise generic measures is the Short Form 36-item Health Survey Questionnaire.[11] This is also often used as a core component to facilitate comparisons across populations in disease-specific batteries of measures. These need to be interviewer administered to obtain the best item response rates among elderly people.[12] In the United States, a commonly used generic scale developed for use with elderly people is the Older Americans' Resources and Services assessment, although the full instrument is lengthy.[13]

Because of the multiple morbidity that is often found in older people, and potential effects on physical functioning, emotional well-being and mental state, most investigators prefer to use a battery of pertinent, domain-specific scales when evaluating the health status or health outcomes of elderly people. These may be used together with relevant, disease-specific or generic measures, while bearing in mind the need to limit respondent fatigue. Popular domain-specific scales include Lawton's Philadelphia Geriatric Center Morale Scale,[14] the Abbreviated Mental Test[15] and the Geriatric Depression Scale.[16] A concise measure of anxiety and depression, which does not include somatic items and is therefore appropriate for use with older people, is the Hospital Anxiety and Depression Scale.[17] The Barthel Index[18] is often used to measure physical functioning, but this is only suitable for severely ill, institutionalised populations. It focuses on self-care at the expense of instrumental tasks of daily living (e.g. domestic tasks) and wider physical mobility. The functioning subsection of the Older Americans' Resources and Services assessment is superior to most scales for use with elderly people.

There is no consensus on recommended batteries of scales. More recently there has been an emphasis on also asking people to list themselves what areas of their life are most important or which have been most affected by their condition. Given that people will have different priorities in life (e.g. the ability to go up a flight of stairs is less important to someone who does not have stairs), these newer instruments provide the means by which individuality can be assessed scientifically.[19,20]

MEASURES OF BROADER QUALITY OF LIFE IN OLDER AGE

The increasing emphasis on evidence-based clinical practice and inclusion of patient-based outcome indicators has led to an increase in the use of health-related and disease-specific measures of quality of life in clinical trials. Interventions which are expected to have a broader impact on a person's life, especially those which enable more independent living at home, also need broader, multidimensional measures of quality of life, and which are relevant to people's lives, for fuller evaluation of outcomes. Three more recent measures of broader quality of life in older age have been developed and tested: the Older People's Quality of Life questionnaire (OPQOL), the CASP-19 measure (domains of Control, Autonomy, Self-realisation and Pleasure) and the World Health Organization Quality of Life Instrument – Older Adults Module (WHOQOL-OLD).

1. The OPQOL was developed bottom-up. Older people's responses to open-ended questioning about the 'good things' that gave life quality were examined. These were categorised into main themes by two researchers, independently. These were, in order of magnitude: social relationships (mentioned by 81%), social roles and activities (60%), solo activities (48%), health (44%), psychological outlook and well-being (38%), home and neighbourhood (37%), financial circumstances (33%) and independence (27%). Smaller numbers mentioned various other things. These responses were consistent with older people's views about what took quality away from life. The themes are detailed in Bowling.[21] The sub-scale domains in the full OPQOL reflect this common core of main constituents of quality of life. The full OPQOL is a 32- to 35-item quality-of-life measure, with the longer version reflecting items also prioritised by ethnically diverse older people in England; it has 5-point Likert scales ranging from 'strongly agree' to 'strongly disagree', with 32 or 35 items, representing life overall (four items); health (four items); social relationships and participation (seven items in quality-of-life follow-up survey, eight items in Omnibus surveys); independence, control over life, freedom (five items); area: home and neighbourhood (four items); psychological and emotional well-being (four items); financial circumstances (four items); religion/culture (two items).[22,23] The measure has been used with geriatric outpatients and was

able to predict their outcomes.[24-26] A short version, OPQOL-brief, has been developed.[27]

2. The CASP-19 measure was developed from the theory of human needs satisfaction, and it was tested with focus groups and a survey of people aged 65–75 years.[28] It concentrates on four theoretically derived domains (19 items): Control (four items), Autonomy (five items), Self-realisation (five items), Pleasure (five items), with 4-point Likert response scales, ranging from 'often' through to 'never'. It has been used in several large population surveys, including the English Longitudinal Study of Ageing.[29]

3. The WHOQOL-OLD was developed from the parent instrument, the World Health Organization's WHOQOL-100, and cross-cultural studies; it was tested on convenience samples of older people across cultures.[30,31] It is a multifaceted measure of quality of life and comprises seven sub-scales (24 items): sensory abilities; autonomy; past, present and future activities; social participation; death and dying; and intimacy (four items per sub-scale). Response scales are 5-point Likert scales and vary in their wording ('not at all' to 'an extreme amount'/'completely'/'extremely'; 'very poor' to 'very good'; 'very dissatisfied' to 'very satisfied'; 'very unhappy' to 'very happy'). The WHOQOL-100 and WHOQOL-OLD have been used with different cultural groups across the world (see www.who.int/mental_health/who_qol_field_trial_1995.pdf).

CRITERIA FOR SCALE DEVELOPMENT AND FOR SELECTING A SCALE

The criteria for measurement scales or batteries of scales are listed in the following paragraphs.[32] When reviewing a scale for use, potential users should check the scale's literature for information on each of these areas, and use an appropriate scale where this information is satisfactory.

Conceptual and measurement model

The conceptual and empirical basis for combining multiple items into a single scale score(s) should be provided. Descriptive statistics for each scale should be provided by scale developers (frequencies, means, central tendency and dispersion, skewness and frequency of missing data), as should procedures for weighting and scoring.

Reliability

The instrument should be free from random error and therefore homogenous in content (high correlations between items and tests of internal consistency). It should be reproducible over time (where changes in scores are not expected) and between raters at one point in time. Scale developers should provide a clear description of the methods used to test for reliability, by type of population, and information on the results of tests for reliability.

Validity

This is the degree to which an instrument measures what it purports to measure. The scale developer should provide evidence that the content of the scale is appropriate and relevant to its intended use, that its construct is sound and that it correlates with measures with which it is theoretically expected to correlate, and that it correlates with a criterion measurement ('gold standard'). As with reliability, full details of the methods, samples and results of tests of validity should be provided by the developer.

Responsiveness

This is the sensitivity of the instrument to true change (e.g. in the patient's condition). This is assessed in before/after studies of interventions and a comparison of scale scores. Assessment of responsiveness involves estimation of the effect size. This is an estimate of the magnitude of change in health status, and it translates the before/after changes into a standard unit of measurement. Scale developers should provide information on responsiveness from longitudinal study data on clearly defined populations.

Interpretability

This is the degree to which meaning can be assigned to the scale's scores. It can be provided by comparative data on the distribution of scores in different populations and on the relationship of scores to clinically recognised conditions and outcomes (including predictive ability of the score in relation to death). The scale developer should provide details of the populations to whom the scale was administered and descriptive statistics.

Burden

Respondent burden can be defined as the time, energy and other demands placed on the respondents during the completion of the instrument. Administrative burden is the demand placed on those who administer it. Developers should not place undue strain on the respondent during the completion of their instruments, and should provide information on average completion times, comprehension or reading levels required, interviewer training required, and the acceptability of the instrument (e.g. indicated by the level of missing data and refusal rates plus reasons).

Alternative forms

These include all of the modes of administration of an instrument, such as self-completion, observer ratings, and interviewer-administered and computer-assisted completion. Evidence of reliability, validity, responsiveness, interpretability and burden should be provided for each form of the instrument.

Cultural and language adaptations

The scale developer should provide information about the conceptual equivalence (equivalence of relevance and meaning of the same concepts) and linguistic equivalence (equivalence of question wording and meaning in the formulation of items, response choices) of the scale in the different languages and repeat the evaluations of its measurement properties (reliability, validity, responsiveness, interpretability and burden). The scale developer should provide evidence of the methods used to achieve equivalence – for example, assessment within each cultural or language group to which the instrument will be applied; two forward translations from the source language by experienced translators and health status research, resulting in a pooled forward translation; back-translations to the source language, resulting in a pooled back-translation; and review of translations by lay and expert panels, with revisions and field-testing to provide evidence of comparability and explanation of any differences.

These criteria should be used to evaluate the strengths and weaknesses of measurement instruments. A wide range of generic and disease-specific measurement scales were concisely reviewed by Bowling in 2001[12] and 2005.[33]

KEY POINTS

- People themselves are the best judges of an outcome of 'life worth living'.
- The only way to address an ethical dilemma about treatment is to ask the patient about his or her perception of his or her quality of life and about his or her preferences.
- If the patient is not competent to answer this question, then ask his or her next of kin or carer who knows the patient best.
- In the ward setting, quality of life may have to be assessed after taking into account the views of the patient and his or her carers with regard to the patient's morale, symptoms, physical dependency, mental capacity and whether he or she is incontinent.
- Although there is no consensus on the recommended battery of scales, commonly used instruments include Lawton's Philadelphia Geriatric Center Morale Scale, the Abbreviated Mental Test and the Geriatric Depression Scale.
- Interventions that have a broad impact on a person's life, especially in the community, may benefit from evaluations using broader measures of quality of life, such as the Older People's Quality of Life questionnaire, the CASP-19 measure (domains of Control, Autonomy, Self-realisation and Pleasure) and the World Health Organization Quality of Life Instrument – Older Adults Module.

REFERENCES

1. McNeil BJ, Weichselbaum R, Pauker SG. Fallacy of the five-year survival in lung cancer. *N Engl J Med.* 1978; **299**(25): 1397–401.
2. McNeil BJ, Weichselbaum R, Pauker SG. Speech and survival: tradeoffs between quality and quantity of life in laryngeal cancer. *N Engl J Med.* 1981; **305**(17): 982–7.
3. Slevin ML, Stubbs L, Plant HJ, *et al.* Attitudes to chemotherapy: comparing views of

patients with cancer with those of doctors, nurses, and general public. *BMJ.* 1990; **300**(6737): 1458–60.

4. Bowling A, Culliford L, Smith D, *et al.* What do patients really want? Patients' preferences for treatment for angina. *Health Expect.* 2008; **11**(2): 137–47.

5. Liddle J, Gilleard C, Neil A. Elderly patients' and their relatives' views on CPR [letter]. *Lancet.* 1993; **342**(8878): 1055.

6. Bowling A, Bond M, McKee D, *et al.* Equity in access to exercise tolerance testing, coronary angiography, and coronary artery bypass grafting by age, sex and clinical indications. *Heart.* 2001; **85**(6): 680–6.

7. Collinson J, Bakhai A, Flather MD, *et al.* The management and investigation of elderly patients with acute coronary syndromes without ST elevation: an evidence-based approach? Results of the Prospective Registry of Acute Ischaemic Syndromes in the United Kingdom (PRAIS-UK). *Age Ageing.* 2005; **34**(1): 61–6.

8. Walter PJ, Mohan R, Amsel BJ. Quality of life after heart valve replacement. *J Heart Valve Dis.* 1992; **1**: 34–41.

9. Bowling A, Gabriel Z, Dykes J, *et al.* Let's ask them: a national survey of definitions of quality of life and its enhancement among people aged 65 and over. *Int J Aging Hum Dev.* 2003; **56**(4): 269–306.

10. Elder AT. Which benchmarks for age discrimination in acute coronary syndrome? *Age Ageing.* 2005; **34**(1): 4–5.

11. Ware JE, Snow KK, Kosinski M, *et al. SF-36 Health Survey: manual and interpretation guide.* Boston, MA: The Health Institute, New England Medical Center; 1993.

12. Bowling A. *Measuring Disease: a review of disease-specific quality-of-life measurement scales.* 2nd ed. Buckingham: Open University Press; 2001.

13. Fillenbaum GG, Smyer MA. The development, validity, and reliability of the OARS Multidimensional Functional Assessment Questionnaire. *J Gerontol.* 1981; **36**(4): 428–34.

14. Lawton MP. The Philadelphia Geriatric Center Morale Scale: a revision. *J Gerontol.* 1975; **30**(1): 85–9.

15. Hodkinson HM. Evaluation of a mental test score for assessment of mental impairment in the elderly. *Age Ageing.* 1972; **1**(4): 233–8.

16. Yesavage JA, Brink TL, Rose TL, *et al.* Development and validation of a geriatric depression screening scale: a preliminary report. *J Psychiatr Res.* 1982–83; **17**(1): 37–49.

17. Zigmond AS, Snaith RP. The Hospital Anxiety and Depression Scale. *Acta Psychiatr Scand.* 1983; **67**(6): 361–70.

18. Mahoney FI, Barthel DW. Functional evaluation: the Barthel Index. *Md State Med J.* 1965; **14**: 61–5.

19. O'Boyle CA, McGee H, Hickey A, *et al.* Reliability and validity of judgement analysis as a method for assessing quality of life. *Br J Clin Pharmacol.* 1989; **27**: 155.

20. Bowling A. The effects of illness on quality of life: findings from a survey of households in Great Britain. *J Epidemiol Community Health.* 1996; **50**(2): 149–55.

21. Bowling A. *Ageing Well: quality of life in older age.* Maidenhead: Open University Press; 2005.

22. Bowling A. The psychometric properties of the Older People's Quality of Life Questionnaire, compared with the CASP-19 and the WHOQOL-OLD. *Curr Gerontol Geriatr Res.* 2009; **2009**: 298950. Epub 2010 Feb 1.

23. Bowling A, Stenner P. Which measure of quality of life performs best in older age? A

comparison of the OPQOL, CASP-19 and WHOQOL-OLD. *J Epidemiol Community Health*. 2011; **65**(3): 273–80. Epub 2010 Aug 18.

24. Bilotta C, Bowling A, Nicolini P, *et al*. Quality of life in older outpatients living alone in the community in Italy. *Health Soc Care Community*. 2012; **20**(1): 32–41. Epub 2011 Jul 1.

25. Bilotta C, Bowling A, Nicolina P, *et al*. Older People's Quality of Life (OPQOL) scores and adverse health outcomes at a one-year follow-up. A prospective cohort study on older outpatients living in the community in Italy. *Health Qual Life Outcomes*. 2011; **9**: 72.

26. Bilotta C, Bowling A, Casè A, *et al*. Dimensions and correlates of quality of life according to frailty status: a cross-sectional study on community-dwelling older adults referred to an outpatient geriatric service in Italy. *Health & Quality of Life Outcomes*, 2010; **8**: 56. Open access. doi:10.1186/1477-7525-8-56

27. Bowling A, Hankins M, Windle G, *et al*. A short measure of quality of life in older age: the performance of the brief Older People's Quality of Life questionnaire (OPQOL-brief). *Arch Gerontol Geriatr*. 2013; **56**(1): 181–7. Epub 2012 Sep 19.

28. Hyde M, Wiggins RD, Higgs P, *et al*. A measure of quality of life in early old age: the theory, development and properties of a needs satisfaction model (CASP-19). *Aging Ment Health*. 2003; **7**(3): 186–94.

29. Blane D, Netuvell G, Montgomery SM. Quality of life, health and physiological status and change at older ages. *Soc Sci Med*. 2008; **66**(7): 1579–87.

30. Power M, Harper A, Bullinger M; WHO Quality of Life Group. The World Health Organization WHOQOL-100: tests of the universality of quality of life in 15 different cultural groups worldwide. *Health Psychol*. 1999; **18**(5): 495–505.

31. Power M, Quinn K, Schmidt S; WHOQOL-OLD Group. Development of the WHOQOL-OLD module. *Qual Life Res*. 2005; **14**(10): 2197–214.

32. Bowling A. *Research Methods in Health*. Maidenhead: Open University Press, in press due 2014.

33. Bowling A. *Measuring Health: a review of quality-of-life measurement scales*. 3rd ed. Buckingham: Open University Press; 2005.

CHAPTER 17

Ethical issues and expenditure on health and social care

Steven Luttrell

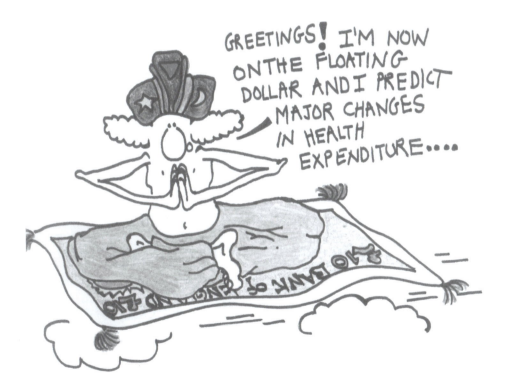

THE NATIONAL HEALTH SERVICE

In the early part of the twentieth century, medical services in the UK were spread unevenly and the National Insurance Scheme did not cover large numbers of poor people. The National Health Service (NHS) was established to provide equitable healthcare provision according to need, irrespective of wealth or geographical location. Over time, it became increasingly clear that comprehensive care, free at the point of delivery, was politically unsustainable. Prescription charges were introduced in 1951, and charges for ophthalmic and dental treatments were introduced thereafter. One of the most radical assaults on the provision of comprehensive care was the shedding by the NHS of substantial parts of its previously held responsibilities for continuing care. In 1982, the NHS was providing 75% of long-stay care for people aged 75 years and over. In 1996 this was reduced to just 18%. During the same time period the population of people aged 75 years and over increased by 25%.

HEALTHCARE OR SOCIAL CARE

The starting point for any discussion on the economics of healthcare in the UK must be a consideration of the meaning of the term 'healthcare'. To define certain care needs as social rather than health related transfers the funding of such services from the NHS (where, in general, costs are provided for by central government) to social services (where, in general, costs are means tested). Although there are many areas of care that are agreed to fall clearly within the remit of the health service, there are others where this is not so obvious. For example, there has been substantial debate over which aspects of continuing care of people with disabilities should be regarded as healthcare and which should be regarded as social care. This debate was set on a legal footing in *R v North and East Devon Health Authority ex part Coughlan* [2000] 3 All ER 850, which clarified the responsibilities of both health and social care services in the provision of longer-term care for people with disabilities and continuing healthcare needs.

PRINCIPLES FOR RATIONING

No matter how narrowly healthcare is defined, there remains a widespread belief that demand for services exceeds supply, and that some form of rationing or prioritisation is necessary. Rationing of healthcare is by no means a new concept. Clinicians have for many decades managed to ration their services implicitly according to unwritten rules. Broadly speaking, healthcare has in the past been rationed according to need, ability to benefit, age and desert.

Need

The allocation of funds according to need has been a traditional function of the NHS. Initial formulas based on mortality ratios were used as proxies for need in order to redistribute funds. Empirical data have led to new formulas that are thought to be more sensitive to the influence of socio-economic factors on health, and which have been applied to the greater part of the NHS budget. However, it has been suggested that the marginal increase in equity associated with the use of the more recent formulas is probably very small, and that in future attention should be focused on the distribution of resources at local levels. Moreover, the allocation of funds according to need does not necessarily mean that such funds will confer benefit.

Ability to benefit

Utilitarian philosophy suggests that funds should be used to provide maximum benefit and the NHS Executive has indicated that resources should increasingly be channelled towards those interventions that are known to be effective.[1] However, while the amount of data on effectiveness continues to rise, only a minority of interventions provided by the NHS are backed by scientific evidence that they confer benefit, and cost–benefit analysis has been applied to even fewer. The complexity of the analysis of data on cost-effectiveness is substantial and health services have been tardy in implementing changes in response to new scientific evidence.

With this in mind, the National Institute for Clinical Excellence (NICE) was established in 1999 to evaluate the clinical and cost-effectiveness of selected new technologies and to make recommendations to the NHS. If NICE ruled in favour of a new product it became mandatory for NHS trusts to provide it. Trusts have also used negative NICE guidance to ration the use of products that are not cost-effective. Although generally perceived as a rationing body, NICE has probably increased NHS expenditure on drugs substantially. It has been criticised for concentrating on new and expensive drugs and its rationing thresholds have been thought by many to be high. Its decisions to restrict access to new treatments continue to be controversial and are challenged by both industry and patient groups.

The Nuffield Council on Bioethics recently suggested the use of minimum effectiveness thresholds as a tool for rationing, arguing that this would be a fair system for rationing care and may be acceptable to both the public and healthcare professionals.

The use of programme budgets is an example of a local systematic approach to reducing waste, reducing unwarranted variations, and improving resource allocation. The approach uses cost and efficacy comparisons between healthcare economies to drive down cost while at the same time improving output. Its focus is local and it may be a more effective method of encouraging the spread of innovative and cost-effective practice than centrally driven systems.

Age

In the past, healthcare has been extensively rationed by age, and there is evidence that older people have been discriminated against with regard to renal replacement therapy, cardiological interventions and cancer treatments. A variety of reasons have been proposed to justify or explain this position.
1. It has been assumed that the needs of older people were somehow less important and that they would not, in any event, benefit from aggressive medical treatment. However, there has been increasing scientific evidence that older people benefit from many medical interventions to which they would previously have been denied access (e.g. treatment of hypertension,

thrombolysis for both myocardial infarction and stroke, carotid artery surgery and renal replacement therapy). In many instances it has been demonstrated that those populations at highest risk of death or complications are often the groups that benefit most from interventions. Thus in certain situations older patients, who are at a greater risk of death or morbidity than younger patients, benefit more from medical treatment.

2. It has been suggested that a strictly utilitarian method of allocating resources discriminates against older people. If it is assumed that the prime function of the NHS is to maximise health, and the 'quality-adjusted life year' is used as a method of assessing outcome, then it becomes obvious that older people, with a shorter life expectancy, will generally rank lower on the priority list than younger people. NICE has been criticised by some for placing a heavy reliance on the use of quality-adjusted life years in its evaluations.

   Harris[2] argues against such a method of distributing resources, stating that patients want the opportunities to have the best possible combination of quantity and quality of life available to them, given their personal health status. It may be valid to use outcome measures when choosing between rival therapies, but this system should not be used for allocating resources between different groups of patients. Harris[2] believes that it is an integral part of distributive justice that people's moral claims to resources are not diminished by who they are (how young or old, rich or poor, powerful or weak they are) or by the quality of their lives. He argues that if the purpose of the NHS is to give people the services that they want for themselves, they would be unlikely to choose the utilitarian approach. This argument has widespread appeal.

3. It is argued by some that the older you are, the more likely you are to have had your 'fair innings', and that it would be inequitable to deny a younger person benefit in order to provide benefit for an older person. According to one view, the fair innings argument is based on the concept of an ideal life and the notion that individuals themselves reach a point in time when they have done all that they would have wished and feel that it is appropriate that they should now die. Although this is an argument that underpins the need for a system where patient autonomy is respected, it adds little to the debate about rationing healthcare.

   According to another view, it is argued that resources should be rationed on the basis of the quality and length of life that any individual has already had. Those who have already had sufficient life of sufficient quality are of lower priority than those who have not. But how can one measure the total quality of any life and how should one decide where the cut-off point for a fair innings should be? A simpler approach has been to argue that resources should be rationed only according to the length of life that an individual has already had. This approach has popular appeal, as evidenced by the frequent media items concerning the plight of babies and children. However, it does highlight basic questions about the value that society attaches to any particular group of individuals. It might be that, despite popular appeal, to stigmatise and undervalue older people in favour of the young is detrimental to the fabric of society as a whole, especially a society that is founded on democratic principles where the value of one person is cherished as much as that of any other. The increasing political power of older people alongside the development of human rights law has done much in recent years to change society's attitude to age.

Within the UK, the most explicit steps to remove rationing on the basis of age were taken initially with the introduction of the National Service Framework for Older People and more recently as a result of the Equality Act 2010. Published in 2001, the first standard of the National Service Framework set out a commitment and listed steps to remove ageism from health and social welfare decisions. The Equality Act 2010 came into force in 2012, making age discrimination unlawful in the provision of services and in the exercise of public functions. The Act covers the provision of all services to the public. While there are some exceptions, there is no express exception in relation to health and social care services. Any age-related differentiated treatment in the provision of health or social care has to be assessed against the objective justification test set out in the Act – that is, is the differentiation a proportionate means of achieving a legitimate aim? The test is has two stages: (i) is the aim of the rule or practice both legal and non-discriminatory, and one that represents a real, objective consideration? and (ii) if the aim is legitimate, is the means of achieving it proportionate – that is, appropriate and necessary in all the circumstances? Is there a less discriminatory approach that could be taken instead? A legitimate aim might be one that has a socially positive outcome or one that is generally in the public interests. For example, an age-based screening service can be justified if it is supported by a statistical analysis of benefit and the approach is seen as a proportionate response to that analysis.

Desert

Giving less to those who are to blame for their illness has an instant emotional appeal. However, as a method for rationing healthcare it is flawed. It is very difficult to draw up a list of those illnesses to which a voluntary choice of lifestyle has contributed. Although alcoholism and cigarette smoking cause a host of illnesses, it is arguable that neither are purely voluntary activities. If cigarette smoking is to be regarded as worthy of moral blame, then is eating an unhealthy diet to be similarly considered? Moreover, although the allocation of moral blame may fall within the responsibility of a legal system, it is questionable whether such judgements fall within the remit of a health service.

HUMAN RIGHTS ACT 1998

There have been several legal cases in England that have considered the implications of the Human Rights Act 1998 and whether this gives patients a right to treatment. The following examples demonstrate the difficulties associated with using this Act as a tool to enforce decisions to fund medical treatments.

➤ Decided in 1999 before the Act came into force in 2000, the Court of Appeal in *North West Lancashire Health Authority v A, D&G*[3] concluded that a refusal to fund gender reassignment surgery did not constitute a breach of article 3 of the Convention on Human Rights (which provides that no one should be subject to inhumane and degrading treatment), and that article 8 (which protects respect for individuals' private lives, including their physical and psychological integrity) does not give a right to treatment. Although this case considered the convention, it is likely that a similar approach would be taken now that the Act is in force.

➤ In 2011 the Court of Appeal in *R v North Staffordshire Primary Care Trust*,[4] in a case concerning bariatric surgery, accepted the primary care trust's (PCT's) submission that the decision not to fund bariatric surgery for the patient did not engage the positive elements of article 8 and was therefore outside a European Court of Human Rights challenge and that the PCT's individual funding policy was justifiable under the Act.

➤ In 2011 the Court of Appeal in *R v Berkshire West Primary Care Trust*,[5] in a case concerning breast augmentation for a transsexual patient, supported the PCT's decision not to fund treatment and rejected an argument that has been supported by the Equality and Human Rights Commission, that the PCT was not entitled to make comparisons between the circumstances of a transsexual and those of a natural woman who suffered psychological distress as a result of lack of breast tissue.

INTERNATIONAL MECHANISMS FOR RATIONING HEALTHCARE

A number of countries have taken steps to develop explicit guidelines about allocating health resources. Many have rejected a strictly utilitarian approach whereby services are ranked according to cost–benefit analysis.

The Swedish Commission stated that such considerations of efficiency should be limited to choices between different kinds of treatment for the same condition, and should not be invoked in the choice between claims for different services or specialties. It highlighted that all people have the same rights irrespective of their personal characteristics, resources should be devoted to those in greatest need and the most vulnerable groups should be given special consideration.

The Dunning Committee in the Netherlands recommended that all claims have to pass four tests:
1. Is the intervention necessary to allow the individual to function in society?
2. Is the treatment effective?
3. Is the treatment efficient?
4. Could the treatment be considered a matter of individual responsibility?

In New Zealand, resource constraints are expressly recognised in the funding framework, the New Zealand Public Health and Disability Act 2000, the objectives of which include a population health focus, community participation and access to appropriate, effective and timely services.

Probably the most adventurous project for rationing healthcare evolved in the state of Oregon in the United States. Like every other US state, it had previously provided only the poorest citizens with Medicaid and left a large percentage of the population unable to use medical services. The Oregon Health Plan was created in 1989 to expand coverage to citizens who at the time had no health insurance. However, in order to fund this expansion the state decided to ration healthcare in a transparent manner by introducing a prioritised list of treatments. A commission was set up to develop this list and heard evidence from both laypeople and professionals. A line was drawn on the list based on the amount of money the state has set aside for its health plan. Everything above the line was covered but those treatments below the line were not. While the plan was initially viewed as successful and the numbers of uninsured people fell, conflicts arose between the state and federal government around the cuts caused by continually raising the 'line'. Moreover, the approach failed to control costs associated with the provision of those treatments above the line. While initial success in reducing uninsured rates was reported, rates during the 2000s rose to levels comparable to the US as whole prompting further reform of the plan including changes to increase screening rates, expand coverage to more children and contain costs by the introduction of premiums and copayments.[6]

Rudolph Klein[7] has suggested that the international principles on which there is agreement are too general to provide any assistance to those who are trying to create a core health service, and he states that rationing by such means has a trivial effect. He believes instead that the reality of rationing is the numerous day-to-day decisions made by clinicians in the light of available resources and the circumstances of the patients before them.

The UK government has not taken steps to define in explicit terms the principles that should be used to ration healthcare, appearing to rely instead on the development of policy from various NHS quality initiatives in combination with the accumulated decisions of healthcare trusts and individual clinicians. Much media and political attention has been paid to the fact that treatment options appear to differ from one part of the country to another. The mechanisms that have been established to counteract this include the development of national standards through a combination of National Service Frameworks and guidance set out by NICE. At the same time, the government has been keen to devolve responsibility for resource allocation to a local level, and responsibility for the allocation of over 70% of the NHS budget now rests with local commissioning groups. There are inevitable tensions created by a system which sets national standards but expects local financial responsibility. While these tensions were masked by the expansion of the total NHS budget in the early 2000s, the more recent tightening of total health spending has prompted further consideration of the relationship between local and national control.

Reforms enacted by the Health and Social Care Act 2012 created a national NHS Commissioning Board working alongside a large number of local clinical commissioning groups and a clearer separation between the commissioning of NHS and public health services.

KEY POINTS

- The NHS was founded on the principle that it would provide an equitable system of healthcare.
- Narrowing the remit of the NHS has been used as a political method for reducing healthcare expenditure.
- Even if healthcare is defined in narrow terms, there appears to be a substantial financial gap between supply and demand.
- Rationing had traditionally been implicit and based on a variety of factors, such as need, ability to benefit, age, and desert.
- A number of countries have attempted to make explicit the principles that should be used in rationing healthcare.
- In the UK, systems have been introduced over recent years in order to steer service delivery along lines that are backed by evidence of effectiveness.
- There is little international agreement about the most effective and fair methods of resource allocation.

REFERENCES

1. *Commissioning Policy: ethical framework for priority setting and resource allocation.* NHS Commissioning Board, April 2013.
2. Harris J. The rationing debate: maximising the health of the whole community. The case against: what the principal objective of the NHS should really be. *BMJ.* 1997; **314**(7081): 669–72.
3. *North West Lancashire Health Authority* v *A, D&G.* [1999] Lloyds Rep Med 399; [2000] 1 WLR 997.
4. *R (Alexander Condliff)* v *North Staffordshire Primary Care Trust and the Secretary of State.* [2011] EWCA Civ 910.
5. *R (C)* v *Berkshire West Primary Care Trust.* [2011] EWCA Civ 247.
6. Fruits E. *The Oregon Health Plan: a "bold experiment" that failed.* Portland, OR: Cascade Policy Institute, 2010.
7. Klein R. The rationing debate: defining a package of healthcare services the NHS is responsible for. The case against. *BMJ.* 1997; **314**(7079): 506–9.

FURTHER READING

- Alakeson V. Why Oregon went wrong. *BMJ.* 2008; **337**: a2044.
- Buyx AM, Friedrich DR, Schöne-Seifert B. Ethics and effectiveness: rationing healthcare by thresholds of minimum effectiveness. *BMJ.* 2011; **342**: d54.
- Department of Health. *Continuing Care: NHS and local councils' responsibilities.* Health Service Circular/Local Authority Circular. 2001; HSC 2001/015: LAC (2001) 18.

- Department of Health. *National Service Framework for Older People*. London: Department of Health; 2001.
- Doyal L. The rationing debate. Rationing within the NHS should be explicit: the case for. *BMJ*. 1997; **314**(7087): 1114–18.
- Drummond M, Weatherly H, Ferguson B. Economic evaluation of health interventions. *BMJ*. 2008; **337**: a1204.
- Government Committee on Choices in Health Care. *Report*. Rijswijk, the Netherlands: Ministry of Welfare, Health and Cultural Affairs; 1992.
- Government Equalities Office. *Equality Act 2010: banning age discrimination in services; an overview for service providers and customers*. London: GEO; 2012.
- Ham C. Retracing the Oregon trail: the experience of rationing and the Oregon health plan. *BMJ*. 1998; **316**(7149): 1965–9.
- Harris J. Unprincipled QALYs: a response to Cubbon. *J Med Ethics*. 1991; **17**(4): 185–8.
- House of Commons Health Committee. *Priority Setting in the NHS: purchasing. Volume 1*. London: HMSO; 1995.
- Manning J, Paterson J. Prioritization: rationing health care in New Zealand. *J Law Med Ethics*. 2005; **33**: 681–97.
- Maynard A. Distributing healthcare rationing and the role of the physician in the United Kingdom National Health Service. In: Grubb A, Mehlman MJ, editors. *Justice and Health Care: comparative perspectives*. Chichester: John Wiley & Sons; 1995.
- Maynard A. The future role of NICE. *BMJ*. 2010; **341**: c6286.
- Maynard A, Bloor K. Help or hindrance? The role of economics in rationing health care. *Br Med Bull*. 1995; **51**(4): 854–68.
- New B; Rationing Agenda Group. The rationing agenda in the NHS. *BMJ*. 1996; **312**(7046): 1593–601.
- Norheim O, Daniels M, Donaldson C. Rationing, a clinical view, and ethical perspective, an economic view. *BMJ*. 2008; **337**: a1846, 1850, 1872.
- Sheldon TA. Formula fever: allocating resources in the NHS. *BMJ*. 1997; **315**(7114): 964.
- Smith R. The failings of NICE. *BMJ*. 2000; **321**(7273): 1363–4.
- Swedish Parliamentary Priorities Commission. *Priorities in Healthcare*. Stockholm: Ministry of Health and Social Affairs; 1995.

Index

CPD with Radcliffe

You can now use a selection of our books to achieve CPD (Continuing Professional Development) points through directed reading.

We provide a free online form and downloadable certificate for your appraisal portfolio. Look for the CPD logo and register with us at: www.radcliffehealth.com/cpd

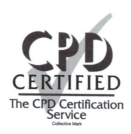

The CPD Certification
Service
Collective Mark